PRIVATE AID, POLITICAL ACTIVISM

PRIVATE AID, POLITICAL ACTIVISM

American Medical Relief to Spain and China, 1936–1949

Aelwen D. Wetherby

UNIVERSITY OF MISSOURI PRESS
Columbia

University of Missouri Press, Columbia, Missouri 65211
Printed and bound in the United States of America
 First printing, 2017

ISBN: 978-0-8262-2107-0
Library of Congress Control Number: 2016960890

∞™ This paper meets the requirements of the
American National Standard for Permanence of Paper
for Printed Library Materials, Z39.48, 1984.

Typefaces: Bembo, Gill Sans

Contents

Abbreviations

ABMAC	American Bureau for Medical Aid to China
AFSC	American Friends Service Committee
AFSD	American Friends of Spanish Democracy
ALB	Abraham Lincoln Brigade
AMBASD	American Medical Bureau to Aid Spanish Democracy
AOA	American Overseas Aid
ARC	American Red Cross
CAC	China Aid Council
CDL	China Defence League
CDS	China Defense Supplies
CLARA	China Liberated Areas Relief Association
CMB	China Medical Board (Rockefeller Foundation)
CNRRA	Chinese National Relief and Rehabilitation Administration
CRC	Chinese Red Cross Society
CSI	*Centrale Sanitaire Internacionale*
EMSTS	Emergency Medical Service Training Schools
FAU	Friends Ambulance Unit
HUAC	House Un-American Activities Committee
ICRC	International Committee of the Red Cross
JAFRC	Joint Anti-Fascist Refugee Committee
MSF	*Médicines Sans Frontières*
PUMC	Peking Union Medical College
SRI	*Socorro Rojo Internacional*
SSI	*Servicio Sanitario Internacional*
UNRRA	United Nations Relief and Rehabilitation Administration
VALB	Veterans of the Abraham Lincoln Brigade
YMCA	Young Men's Christian Association

Archival Abbreviations

NARA	National Archive and Record Administration
HP-FDRL	Hyde Park, Franklin D. Roosevelt Presidential Library
NYPL	New York Public Library

PRIVATE AID, POLITICAL ACTIVISM

An Introduction

In the winter and spring of 1938, the short-lived *Journal of the Association of Medical Students* published a debate between Harvard University physiologist and professor Dr. Walter B. Cannon and National Secretary of the American Red Cross (ARC) Miss Mabel T. Boardman. The question was how to ameliorate modern war with medical aid—and, more specifically, how to do so in light of the civil war that had recently fragmented Spain. Although Cannon and Boardman's discussion offers interesting reflections on concepts of modernity in the mid-twentieth century, something more fundamental was at stake. In the late 1930s, with the embers of smaller conflicts throughout the globe threatening combustion, Cannon and Boardman grappled with how, as self-proclaimed servants of a common global humanity and citizens of the United States, they should serve both national and global communities in responding to the outbreak of war beyond American borders.[1]

Cannon and Boardman proposed two visions of aid drawing from the same language of ethics and action. According to Boardman:

> It may be difficult for those not closely associated with the Red Cross to understand this "spirit of the Treaty of Geneva," referred to in the Congressional Charter. This is the pure spirit of mercy and humanity . . . It is not a judge, but a mitigator of sufferings caused by war or disaster. No physician worthy of his calling would stop to question the moral character of some injured victim of a sudden accident, before rendering the aid his merciful skill could provide . . . The very fact of its singleness of purpose gives to the Red Cross a power almost beyond belief.[2]

Boardman connected the "spirit" of the Red Cross, with the fundamental "spirit" of mercy within the medical profession—a mercy that was above and beyond assessment of moral character. In also connecting Red Cross legitimacy to its relationship to the state, Boardman's claim to legitimacy was exclusive in its "singleness of purpose" and sphere of action. But was the ARC's close connection as a private organization to the machinery of the

U.S. government really unique? With long-standing anti-statist traditions favoring local action over federally organized governance, private entities had long been employed by American policymakers to generate collective action for public purposes.[3] Making out that sphere to be an *international* one did, however, mark a departure from the ARC's pre-war image. Prior to World War I, the ARC's focus had been closely tied to domestic disaster relief. By the end of the war, however, the ARC had emerged as the preeminent U.S. institution involved in international humanitarian relief.

Cannon did not disagree with Boardman's assessment of the ethical commitments of the medical profession in ministering aid to the victims of war. As Cannon summarized, "War, more than any other human experience, puts the medical profession to a supreme test. It is worse than pestilence, for it is almost sure to include pestilence, starvation and the depths of misery, not only among combatants but also among innocent non-combatants."[4] Cannon had served in the medical corps in World War I and, like many of his colleagues, still looked to the years between 1914 and 1918 as setting the standards upon which to base contemporary programs of medical aid.[5] In the 1930s Cannon became involved in the American Medical Bureau to Aid Spanish Democracy (AMBASD), an organization dedicated to offering medical assistance to Republican Spain during the Spanish Civil War. He addressed the partisanship of this group directly:

> The question naturally arises, why not aid both sides? Of course, any wounded brought to our units are humanely treated, whichever side they represent. The ethics of the medical guild requires its members to perform their services to friend and foe alike . . . That is the professional spirit. Why not, then, aid both sides? In a war, differences of attitude are well separated and are likely to be intense. Persons who are at all interested will favor one side or the other. I and persons associated with me in the Medical Bureau sympathize with the legitimate government in Spain, and though we labor with the professional spirit, we apply our main efforts on the side of the government.[6]

Cannon did not question or negate Boardman's spirit of mercy as it would apply to the standards of the medical profession. He did, however, add a layer of moral responsibility that extended into the political realm. Finding "the central struggle of our time . . . dramatized in Spain . . . between democracy, on the one hand, and aggressive dictatorship, on the other," Cannon found his moral responsibility within a more selective application of aid.[7] To actively aid Fascism as a matter of humanitarian policy, by Cannon's estimation, corrupted the ideals that fed the humanitarian impulse. Cannon also cited the legitimacy granted by the state in noting, "We are permitted by the State Department . . . to show our sympathy in caring for the wounded and the innocent victims of the insurrection."[8] For Cannon, becoming a true humanitarian required a political choice beyond neutrality. And he would be joined by many more in this perspective, as private grassroots efforts blended ARC traditions of humanitarian engagement with more consciously political choices.

Using a handful of grassroots organizations founded by concerned Americans, this book will explore American medical relief to Spain and China in the late 1930s and 1940s as responses to the outbreak of the Spanish Civil War (1936–1939) and the Second Sino-Japanese War (1937–1945). I selected these two conflicts because of what, at first, appeared to be a series of direct links and overlapping involvement between the people involved in the AMBASD and private aid to China. Upon further research, however, such linkages proved less significant, but other parallels emerged. Although serving vastly different peoples in strikingly distant landscapes—and set apart by their variable political and social support in the U.S.—the AMBASD, American Bureau for Medical Aid to China (ABMAC), and China Aid Council (CAC) illustrate more than a series of distinct geopolitical responses. Their shared history illustrates a transition in how people responded to foreign conflict and how humanitarian aid was used as a political tool from the interwar period through World War II. Although a substantial secondary literature exists surrounding both the Spanish Civil War and Second Sino-Japanese War—and international involvement in them—historical examinations of these conflicts in tandem remains relatively new, despite parallels in the eyes of their contemporaries.[9]

The people behind this new wave of organizational activity shared a sense of political and social activism that set them apart from other groups. In the U.S., these beliefs led such activists to diverge from broader patterns in the American populace and other established American institutions in responding to foreign wars. For some of these individuals, the Spanish Civil War and the Second Sino-Japanese War presented parallel threats to democratic traditions.[10] For others—many recent immigrants—regional ties to homelands besieged by conflict presented a call to action. These diverse groups shared a dedication to the development of moral and political activism through the means of medicine, a "medical activism" inspired by a belief in the potential of the private citizen to mediate international relations, and the moral responsibility to make political choices in the offer of aid.

This study also seeks to add new detail to the history of U.S. international relations in the 1930s—a period in which there was a constant and growing tension between internationalist and isolationist agendas. With federal foreign policies generally emphasizing the latter, private action became an increasingly relevant alternative route for those interested in international matters. As private citizens sought to become mediators of international relations, the federal government navigated means to manage this private action. As a contribution to the growing body of work moving away from a policy- and government-oriented perspective on international relations to a more multifaceted examination of the totality of interactions among "peoples, organizations, states, and systems," this book offers a snapshot of private international action in the 1930s.[11]

The story of these otherwise small and relatively unknown organizations can help refine historical understanding of the development of humanitarianism and the evolution of global citizenship in the twentieth century. As noted by Akira Iriye, an early proponent for the internationalization of history, "A focus on international organizations, rather than nations and states, as units of analysis provides a fresh perspective on the evolution of international relations and enables us to reconceptualize modern world history."[12] Ian Tyrrell has also demonstrated the potential that lies in the study of smaller organizations to offer a window into much larger trends of American international activity and cultural expansion.[13] Although much of the work of the individuals in this study was still framed in highly nationalistic terms, the men and women discussed here ultimately saw their civic, professional, and patriotic duty as extending beyond U.S. borders. Distinct from peace movements and international action that immediately followed World War I, these groups sought to mediate suffering while simultaneously supporting the basis for the conflicts that triggered their foundation. At the same time, however, the vocabulary of universal humanitarian ideals pervaded the language of these organizations. Faced with the expansion of conflict abroad, how did these individuals strive to maintain such ideals alongside larger geopolitical tensions and choices?

Activists and Humanitarians

Private activism as a response to war was not without historical precedent. There are parallels to be drawn to a long traditional of private volunteerism in war, from medieval crusaders to nineteenth-century filibusterers. An examination of the historical development of the AMBASD, ABMAC, and CAC reveals a shared impulse of responding to crisis through activism, bridging both political and humanitarian ideals. Tracing this evolution also demonstrates the ways in which activist threads of humanitarianism were woven into changing institutional structures of aid, and also how that aid would increasingly be seen as a diplomatic and strategic tool in wielding influence alongside more traditional military aims. In combining traditions of political activism with the outlet of medical relief, I argue that the people of the AMBASD, ABMAC, and CAC became medical activists, seeking to employ the moral imperative of humanitarian assistance to protest American foreign policy and push for more active interventions in foreign conflict just short of war (although even this line at times became hazy). Such humanitarian efforts also gave individuals an outlet for acting on personal ideals during a period in which they felt that their voices were marginalized. Meanwhile, concurrent developments in U.S. foreign policy began to selectively reinforce certain private efforts, illustrating a shift in attitudes toward the potential of humanitarian relief to serve as a mediator of international relations.

However, the idea of "medical activism" differentiates early medical relief efforts to Spain and China from more established international health and welfare activities in a number of ways. Activism not only combines political motives and humanitarian ideals, but also classifies such work as a more spontaneous, grassroots effort. Introducing the concept in describing a collection of letters from American medical volunteers in the Spanish Civil War, Cary Nelson labels their story "the founding moment of modern medical activism . . . because their motivation was not only humanitarian, but also political."[14] Nelson's proposal highlights the critical conflict within contemporary and historical discussions of aid in proposing a distinct separation between the "political" and the "humanitarian." Humanitarian medical relief was often distinguished from other forms of international involvement for its independence from politics. How could one reproach a basic concern for human welfare, based upon the objective scientific realities of modern medicine? In reality, matters were rarely so simple, and the line between political conviction and humanitarian idealism has historically been difficult to define.[15] As observed by Emily S. Rosenberg on early twentieth-century philanthropic activity, "Relief efforts, like other philanthropic impulses, were built on contradictory imagery. Although usually cast in apolitical terms, emergency assistance efforts invariably became entangled in politics—both international politics and those of the relief bureaucracies themselves."[16]

This study does not seek to provide a comprehensive study of organizations at work in either Spain or China, but instead will focus on the development of three: AMBASD, ABMAC, and CAC. As Americans watched war break out in Spain in 1936 and China in 1937, many felt compelled to respond. Despite many differences, the AMBASD (founded in 1936 to aid Republican Spain), the ABMAC (founded in 1937 to aid Nationalist China), and the CAC (founded in 1937 to aid Communist China) shared common qualities in seeking new avenues of applying private aid initiatives.

Focusing on medical relief as a particular strand of humanitarian aid provides a structure for an examination of how political activism may evolve from a grassroots effort to a larger public enterprise. In this sense, despite different trajectories, medical relief efforts to both Spain and China illustrate the extent to which the state recognized private aid as a tool of foreign relations.[17] The organizations of this study, however, were far from the only ones working to aid Spain and China during this period. Many other groups faded in and out of the picture, ranging from similarly small, private efforts, to larger institutions such as the ARC and United Nations Relief and Rehabilitation Administration (UNRRA). Quaker involvement through the American Friends Service Committee (AFSC) also maintained a consistent presence in both Spain and China. Quaker activities have been largely excluded from consideration here, which chooses to focus more on organizations that incorporated more of a political voice into their relief efforts.

As destinations for conscientious objectors to the conflicts of both world wars, the British Friends Ambulance Unit (FAU) and the AFSC provide a philosophical contrast to the organizations of this study. Quaker-affiliated medical relief has been described as one of the few truly neutral conduits to offer any significant aid during the Spanish Civil War.[18] In 1941, the FAU organized the China Convoy, which sent medical volunteers to work alongside the Chinese Red Cross in mobile units.[19] By 1946, the AFSC had joined the effort with 18 American volunteers, although over half of the 139 volunteers still came from Britain.[20] Although some have pointed out that the FAU was never an "official Quaker body," it did provide important work for young pacifists to respond proactively to the devastation of war.[21] When the AFSC became affiliated with UCR, the China Convoy found new support through its American volunteers. For the remaining years of the war, UCR became the China Convoy's principal source of funding, which, combined with a British "grant-in-aid" and help from the Canadian Red Cross, reportedly gave the unit stronger financial backing than any other Quaker group in operation.[22] The work of the FAU in World War II later earned the Quakers a Nobel Peace Prize in 1947. With the roots of Quaker relief efforts in pacifist ideals, perhaps even these efforts may not be considered outside of political aims. But there is a significant distinction between Quaker relief's fundamental opposition to war, in contrast to the implicit acceptance by the AMBASD, ABMAC, and CAC.

Isolationists and Internationalists

With formal U.S. foreign policy set on a course of isolationism from world affairs, and an economic crisis that brought about major changes in American society, culture, and domestic policy, historical research on the 1930s has focused predominantly on these themes. Yet despite overarching domestic concerns, and foreign policy that sought to limit U.S. intervention, there remains an international history to be told.[23] This study seeks to bridge themes of internationalism and domestic change during the 1930s through an examination of how private international activism developed alongside contrasting—and occasionally collaborative—policies on the federal level. But, in considering an international history of the 1930s, can isolationism be dismissed entirely?

During the 1930s, American activity abroad was a matter of debate. But it was less a matter of *whether* the U.S. should engage in the global sphere and more a matter of *how* it should do so. Robert Dallek offers language for a more nuanced approach, presenting political tensions during the administration of President Franklin D. Roosevelt as divided between "internationalists" and "isolationists."[24] Like debates between "imperialists" and "anti-imperialists" at the turn of the century, or those of "interventionists" and "non-interventionists" at the brink of World War II, these dichotomies often crossed traditional political boundaries of the Democratic and Republican parties. As historians have worked to internationalize U.S. history, the limits of isolationism have become increasingly evident.[25] As argued by Cohen, "While the narrative of isolationism implies self-obsessed ignorance and contempt for engagement in world affairs" even advocates of "international peace, justice, arbitration, non-intervention, and anti-imperialism . . . had little to do with isolation but instead represented an alternative yet activist foreign policy paradigm."[26] In Cohen's dichotomy, the organizations that developed in response to the outbreak of war in Spain and China in the late 1930s fell somewhere between these extremes. While seeking to ameliorate the effects of war, many of these agencies espoused an interventionist—and ultimately war-affirming—approach to medical relief.

Acknowledging the greater intricacies present in American interwar political culture, the 1930s saw the political influence of the isolationists in congressional action. Over the course of the decade, U.S. efforts to avoid direct participation in foreign wars became formally articulated in a series of laws collectively known as the Neutrality Acts. At least in part inspired by popular responses to the Nye Committee's findings, Congress passed the first of these on 31 August 1935, prohibiting the export of war materiel from the U.S. to any warring nations.[27] Following the Italian invasion of Ethiopia that fall, the act was renewed and expanded to prohibit Americans from extending loans or credits to belligerents. As private citizens began joining the International Brigades in the Spanish Civil War, the act was renewed and redefined in May 1937 to explicitly include civil war and to prohibit the transport of any passengers or materials to belligerent nations on U.S. ships. U.S. citizens were also prohibited from traveling on ships belonging to belligerent nations. Humanitarian aid was still allowed, although aid organizations had to register for a license from the State Department and submit monthly audits of their activities.[28] However, even within these policies tensions existed, as Roosevelt sought greater executive discretion in applying the Neutrality Acts. He eventually gained a degree of this in the cash-and-carry provision conceded by Congress in the 1939 Act.[29] This provision gave the president the discretion to allow nations at war to acquire any materials in the U.S. except arms, so long as they paid for such items up front and transported them on non-U.S. ships.

In spite of such federal efforts to regulate private action in international affairs, a number of American citizens defied the stipulations of the Neutrality Acts.[30] Nearly 2,800 Americans traveled to Spain to join the International Brigades and fight on behalf of the Spanish Republic. In China, some parallels can be found in the private formation (albeit quietly condoned by the U.S. government) of the American Volunteer Group (AVG), led by retired American colonel Claire Lee Chennault in 1939.[31] When the U.S. entered the war as China's ally, many AVG pilots were absorbed into U.S. Army Air Force's 23rd Fighter Group.[32] Such private efforts became another iteration of ongoing conflicts between private and state action in the international arena.

Americans fighting on behalf of foreign armed forces may have left less room for debate when considered to be in conflict with U.S. foreign policy or national interests. However, in the field of non-military aid, the boundaries proved more difficult to define. And the outbreaks of war in Spain and China were not the first instances of foreign conflict instigating private action of U.S. citizens outside of or in contrast to governmental responses. In 1824, American aid organizations had sprung up out of sympathy for Greece in the

Greek War of Independence. Supporters of Greece sought federal backing in their efforts by urging Congress that supplying the Greeks with food and basic supplies was a simple act of humanitarianism and would not violate neutrality. Ultimately, however, they had to rely solely on private donations for their work.[33] Shortly before the outbreak of war in Spain and China in the 1930s, Americans organized aid for Ethiopia following the start of the

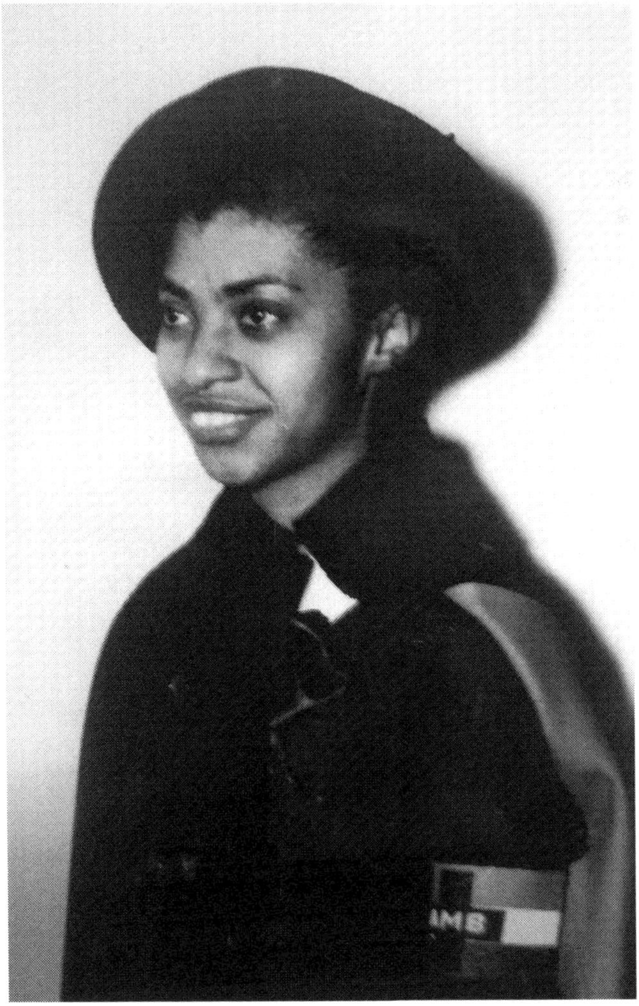

Figure 1. Nurse Salaria Kee (above) was involved in Harlem Hospital's fundraising for Ethiopia before traveling to Spain with the AMBASD. Dentist Arnold Donowa was also involved in both projects (Patai Papers, Tamiment Library, New York University).

Second Italo-Ethiopian War, finding special resonance within the African American community. As United Aid for Ethiopia raised money to provide non-military aid (some of which was sent to the Ethiopian Red Cross), doctors and nurses of Harlem Hospital in New York collected medical supplies and funds to send a seventy-five–bed hospital to Ethiopia.[34] Although ultimately more limited in scope, these activities served as an inspiration for later organizations dedicated to aiding Spain.[35]

In other periods and circumstances, citizen activism became an instigator for and ally to state action. In the aftermath of World War I, numerous private agencies arose to undertake the work of the transition from war to peace. In the U.S., the American Relief Administration (ARA) became an important program pursuing aid with political overtones.[36] Although founded by Congress in 1919, the ARA eventually became a joint public and private venture, with its initial budget of $100 million doubled by private donations. With this support, the ARA delivered more than four million tons of relief supplies to twenty-three European countries. It also offered a popular foundation for ARA Director Herbert Hoover to later serve as U.S. president between 1929 and 1933. The ARC emerged from the war having expanded exponentially and established a new precedent in straddling private and state spheres of action.[37] The interwar period also saw the development of major international societies, such as the League of Red Cross Societies, League of Nations Health Organization, and Rockefeller Foundation's International Health Division.[38]

When Franklin D. Roosevelt assumed the presidency in 1933, his administration worked to clearly define government and private spheres in New Deal action. Under this model, private aid efforts had substantial freedom to develop independently. At the same time, the difficult economic conditions of the Great Depression tested the limits of private aid and contributed to an expansion of state involvement.[39] During this period, missionary-based philanthropic efforts of prior decades were increasingly transformed into formats of more secularized and professionalized aid and institutional development.[40] This study reinforces this general development sequence, while perhaps adding another dimension. Even beyond moving away from religiously inspired aid toward more secular avenues, the organizations of this study may be seen as politicizing that mission. In doing so, these organizations may have laid an unconscious preamble to more recent proclamations of the power of "medical diplomacy."[41]

While marking a new chapter in humanitarian work, interwar humanitarianism still balanced the tensions between international and national interests implicit in the challenge of international aid. As such individuals sought to build the post-war peace and began work in translating sympathy for the victims of war into a new language of rights, transnational networks sought to move beyond national boundaries.[42] Studies of conflict and humanitarian response in the Middle East, in particular, illustrate the extent to which the systems and language of humanitarian work have drawn from unique geographical and interpersonal relationships.[43] As Michelle Tusan has pointed out, "How a humanitarian standard is applied to particular groups at particular moments requires historical explanation."[44]

Numerous studies claim the birth of "modern humanitarianism" to rest in the period following World War I. And, with World War I often marked as the birthplace of total war, the parallel between the new threat posed to private citizens with the activism that followed gains new meaning. But with post-war aid focused on maintaining the peace and preventing future conflict, the wave of organizations considered in this study seem to appear made of a different cloth, even while employing a similar developing language of humanitarian rights. In practice, efforts of a group such as the AMBASD may share more with the ARC during World War I than any post-war aid effort. And across the AMBASD, ABMAC, and CAC, the sense of humanitarian aid being connected to a moral responsibility to *defend* a threatened group ran hand-in-hand with *fighting against* an aggressor. And yet, when it came to the fight itself, groups such as the AMBASD, ABMAC, and CAC, remained one step short of military intervention by remaining immersed in the language of humanitarianism and practice of medical aid.

Building off of the changes that began in the interwar period, World War II became a turning point in the development of humanitarian aid. Various arguments have been proposed for the significance of this watershed in humanitarianism.[45] Speaking less directly to humanitarianism, James Sparrow has emphasized the war's role in restructuring the U.S. government.[46] During a period in which many other countries turned toward constructing the modern welfare state, U.S. mobilization for World War II led to a major break with the aloof tradition of the Monroe Doctrine in international affairs established over a century earlier. Oliver Zunz proposed that after World War II the division established by Roosevelt's New Deal between government and private action became irrelevant, and American philanthropic organizations began increasingly turning their attention to overseas relief and reconstruction.[47] Michael Barnett reinforced the war's role as a turning point between two of his three defined eras of humanitarian history.[48] While proposing a valuable chronological framework for the field, further detail can be added to this framework in examining more of the cultural forces at play.

While World War II certainly proved a turning point, this study emphasizes that the roots of the changes marked by most historians began during the interwar period. The organizations of this study—and the "medical activists" behind them—can be seen as outgrowths of this tradition as well. Preceding the program of aid established by Lend-Lease (which would have ramifications for China, if not for Spain), private aid efforts as described here were intimately tied to war. Although activists often cited ideals of neutrality in ascribing to humanitarian traditions, this was a humanitarianism couched in the assumption that pacifism was not a solution.

American Aid to Spain

The sense of duty to engage in the conflict in Spain was certainly shared by the nearly 2,800 Americans who joined the International Brigades on behalf of the Spanish Second Republic. Although a mythology has developed surrounding the Abraham Lincoln Brigade, very little attention has been paid to the larger efforts to provide non-military aid to Spain that spread through the U.S. and other Western democracies.[49] Eric R. Smith's *Spanish Relief Aid* provides a much-needed analysis of the landscape of American aid efforts in the Spanish Civil War, emphasizing the wide range of social, political, and ethnic groups it involved.[50] Smith limits his discussion to the structure and activities of the aid "movement" within the U.S., and focuses less on their activities in Spain. More gender-oriented studies of women's involvement in the Spanish Civil War also offer a valuable portrait of American nursing personnel, including Julia Newman's 2002 documentary film and Frances Patai's study of American nurses in Spain.[51] Examining medical aid efforts in light of the propaganda they generated, Rey García discusses the inherent contrast between partisan medical aid and the non-partisan humanitarian motives they publicized. She notes that of the dozens of American organizations that sent medical aid to Spain, only seven could be considered neutral—of which only the ARC and Quaker Society of Friends participated in any significant way.[52] More general histories mention aid efforts, but these references usually remain peripheral.[53]

American medical units, however, were ultimately one piece within larger health service structures in Republican Spain. Spanish historians, generally speaking, have done more to emphasize the role of national units as smaller parts of a broadly international effort.[54] This effort not only enlisted the help of medical personnel from dozens of countries, but was also integrated with the work of Spanish medical personnel. Nicolas Coni's comprehensive study of medicine during the Spanish Civil War offers an exception to this general trend, providing an overview of both Nationalist and Republican medical structures and the medical advances made on both sides.[55] Studies on British medical volunteers during the Spanish Civil War are also worth noting as valuable references for piecing together the experience of Americans in Spain and the blurring of national lines that separated different national volunteer units in Spain.[56] Although national medical units operated relatively independently, volunteers from different countries often worked together at different facilities.

Although the AMBASD was founded separately, its units and volunteers became closely affiliated with the American contingent of the International Brigades. For many of the veterans of the Abraham Lincoln Brigade, like the volunteers of the AMBASD, the experience of Spain became part of a larger life of political activism. Peter Carroll has argued that for the majority of American veterans, participation in the Spanish Civil War arose more from shared working-class political beliefs and concerns over the rise of Fascism, than from manipulation by the Comintern and American Communist Party.[57] Carroll mentions some of the more prominent medical volunteers as part of his study, but does not provide a comprehensive account of volunteer medical units.[58] Dialogues over the political components of relief work in Spain fit into a much larger historical debate over the role of the Communist involvement in the Spanish Civil War. In the U.S., this debate became particularly volatile with the emergence of the Cold War and the rise of McCarthyism after World War II. Such debates would not, however, be isolated to the aid of Spain.

American Aid to China

When the Spanish Civil War ended in 1939, the AMBASD faded away, leaving its supporters to seek new avenues of professional and political action. However, with the approach of World War II, the private initiatives of the ABMAC and the CAC began to take off. In 1941, both groups (alongside six other private aid agencies) were incorporated under the auspices of United China Relief, Inc. (UCR).[59] In the six years following its foundation, UCR and its member agencies collected nearly $50 million in aid, at least $10 million of which was dedicated to the medical activities of the ABMAC.[60] UCR also acquired an impressive list of supporters, including Pearl S. Buck, J.D. Rockefeller III, Colonel Theodore Roosevelt, Wendell L. Willkie, Mayling Soong, Eleanor Roosevelt, and Henry R. Luce.[61] Luce's role, in particular, has drawn attention in studies of UCR's impact on American attitudes toward China, and references to UCR have been included in numerous histories of Sino-American relations in the mid-twentieth century.[62] In 1942, the Chinese ambassador presented medals of honor to six American doctors for their efforts to provide aid to China through the ABMAC.[63] As the leading UCR agency in the field of medical relief, the ABMAC has received comparatively scant historical attention.[64] The CAC, also active in the medical field under UCR leadership, has received even less.

Although both sought to promote China's cause through medical aid, the ABMAC and CAC drew from different American bases of support. Outside of Chinese-American communities, ABMAC leadership drew heavily from networks established through the Rockefeller Foundation's China Medical Board and American missionary groups. Through the China Medical Board's Peking Union Medical College (PUMC), an international community of physicians and academics developed, as educational exchanges encouraged movement and communication between Chinese and American medical students and faculty.[65]

Many physicians involved in these exchanges had prior experience with China through American missionary efforts. The same was true of many early supporters and leaders of these private groups. Both UCR president Luce and UCR board member Pearl S. Buck were "mishkids," born in China to missionary parents and profoundly affected by their early experience in China.[66] Dr. Walter Judd, a former medical missionary in China involved in the Student Volunteer Movement, later became a U.S. congressman and active member of UCR. Judd's political life, informed by his experiences in China, also led him to be an influential member of the "China lobby" speaking vehemently against the Chinese Communists' rise to power.[67] While the religious dimensions of the Nationalist and Communist divide led many with missionary ties to identify with the Nationalist government, others ended up becoming strong supporters of the Communists in China.[68] For others, such as Dr. Ruth Hemenway, ideological motivations remained a secondary priority to professional objectives.[69]

While the ABMAC tended to draw more from missionary and Rockefeller Foundation communities, the China Aid Council (CAC) found many supporters among those active in providing medical aid to the Spanish Republic. CAC executive secretary, Marian Exter, first gained organizational experience working with the AMBASD. The CAC provided support to the network of International Peace Hospitals in the Northwest, which Canadian surgeon and Spanish Civil War medical veteran Dr. Norman Bethune played an important role in establishing.[70] American physician Dr. George Hatem adopted a leading role in China's International Peace Hospitals during the war.[71] China also became the destination for a number of refugee doctors from central and eastern Europe, with many finding politically sympathetic colleagues among the Chinese Communists, with a handful also serving with U.S. military forces in Nationalist war zones.

Meanwhile, UCR's relationship with the U.S. government continued to develop, and from 1943 onward, the vast majority of UCR's funding came from the National War Fund. Announced in 1943 by President Roosevelt with his hearty approval, the National War Fund was established to offer American citizens "a share in winning the war, and in winning the right of free men to live in a better world" and to demonstrate to America's allies that they had "the backing of all the resources and spirit of the American people themselves."[72] Ultimately, however, the entrance of the U.S. into World War II and the growth of larger governmental initiatives ultimately eclipsed smaller private aid efforts to China in terms of financial impact. This period also saw significant changes in federal structures for accommodating—and overseeing—private humanitarian initiatives.[73]

A Note on Sources

This study draws extensively from archival sources, offering new detail to previously untold stories. With much of my research on the AMBASD drawing from Fredericka Martin's research into the organization during the 1960s and 1970s, inspired by her own work as head nurse of the first AMBASD unit, this study will undoubtedly have been colored by her own interests. At the same time, Martin's collection offers a unique resource in gathering material on people who otherwise do not appear often in the historical record—and in gaining invaluable perspectives of personal reflection. Supplementing her work with those of other relevant collections in the Tamiment Archives of New York University and secondary sources coming from both Spain and the U.S., I have tried to draw conclusions from echoes across multiple sources. While vast organizational collections exist for the ABMAC and UCR, very little archival resources remain surrounding the CAC. Future research into the China Defence League in China may reveal new sources relevant to this study, if any archival materials still exist. Without the equivalent of a Fredericka Martin, following up with volunteers after the war, the voices and biographical details of those involved in American aid to China have been more difficult to track down. Additionally, perspectives of Chinese recipients of aid have been largely absent from the resources currently available.

With much of this book's priorities lying in bringing archival material to light, I hope it may pave the way for supplementary research in the future. As a study in U.S. political activism, a broader look at citizen action in response to the wars of the 1930s—beyond medical relief—would offer another interesting story at this chapter in history. Alternatively, remaining within the realm of medical relief and humanitarian aid, including an examination of private American responses to the Italo-Ethiopian War would be an interesting addendum. In his work, Eric R. Smith has hinted at connections between Spain and the Ethiopian aid movements, noting that in early 1937 the Communist Party sought to redirect aid collected for Ethiopia to Spain, with the slogan that "Ethiopia's fate is at stake on the battlefields of Spain."[74] These three major conflicts, all leading up to World War II, compose an important trajectory in American interwar history, driving both the more formal statements of American foreign policy claimed in the Neutrality Acts of the 1930s, and other responses—such as those examined in this study—working to circumvent or confront those policies.

Outline of Chapters

The first half of this study will examine the foundation and development of the AMBASD, ABMAC, and CAC within their U.S. context. More specifically, Chapter 1 will provide a closer examination of the people behind the efforts of these organizations and the motivations behind and rationale for their action. All three organizations were founded on a remarkably similar timeline, following the outbreak of the Spanish Civil War in July 1936, and the Second Sino-Japanese War in July 1937 by a several months. Chapter 2 further develops the idea of "medical activism" as a trend in private aid that contrasted with more established institutions, such as the ARC. Critical of the perceived lack of an appropriate ARC response, organizations such as the AMBASD, ABMAC, and CAC began to supplant the traditionally neutral role of the ARC in foreign medical relief by more directly embracing the political dimensions of humanitarian aid. Chapter 3 offers a closer examination of how each of these organizations began to expand, particularly in light of changing federal structures. Beginning as smaller grassroots responses spearheaded, at least in the case of the AMBASD and the ABMAC, by medical personnel with distinctive political beliefs (the CAC's exact origins are murkier), all three evolved to become a part of larger federated aid efforts. In the case of Spain, the North American Committee sought to unite a number of relief responses that had formed in response to the war in Spain. In the case of China, United China Relief (UCR) became the uniting force behind an even greater diversity of aid efforts, which included both the ABMAC and the CAC. Meanwhile, the U.S. government moved toward recruiting private efforts seen to be supportive of U.S. interests in foreign policy. A closer examination of evolving federal attitudes toward private aid reflects the extent to which private success still relied on alignment with state interests.

The second half of this study turns its attention toward Spain and China to explore the activities of each these organizations abroad. Chapter 4 will examine the activities of the AMBASD in Spain, while Chapter 5 will focus on those of the ABMAC and the CAC in China. This section seeks to draw attention to different levels of humanitarian action by focusing on the experiences of the medical volunteers and logistical representatives that translated organizational policy and ideals to reality in the field. This individualized approach offers a unique perspective in considering some of the more tangible impacts of these organizations. Chapter 6 returns focus to the U.S. in order to view how the political dimensions—and political controversies—of such aid efforts began to turn a former strength into a destructive force. This book examines the complex interplay between private and state interests. Both influenced and depended on one other, as private organizations and state bodies sought to maintain autonomy and control. The organizations that ultimately found the greatest financial success were those that ran in tandem with U.S. state interests. Finally, this study will conclude by offering a consideration of how the private efforts described fitted into the larger trajectory of humanitarian medical relief in the twentieth century, and how medical activism contributed to the institutionalization of medical diplomacy.

CHAPTER ONE

Americans Respond
The Development of Private Aid

Although the Spanish Civil War and Second Sino-Japanese War were products of unique geopolitical circumstances, both became linked in the rise of conflict in the interwar world. In Britain, this connection became framed as the "Shanghai-Madrid axis."[1] Both conflicts resonated with one another, not only as combats over Fascist power or imperialist aggression, but also in turning civilians into new targets of conflict. In the U.S., parallel public responses arose. The bombing of civilian centers from Bilbao and Madrid to Shanghai and Nanking were cited in parallel as evidence of the new realities of war.[2] And yet, as news of the aerial bombardment of civilian centers marched across pages of both British and American newspapers, the governments of both remained firm in official policies of nonintervention. Popular dissent against these policies, coupled with a sense of sympathy and moral obligation toward those mired in the conflicts themselves, laid the foundation for the development of private aid initiatives to assist causes in both Spain and China.

The stories of organizations such as the AMBASD, ABMAC, and the CAC, reveal the more complex story behind the destinations of aid. Arising out of sympathies for a particular side of each conflict (and sometimes smaller factions within one side of one conflict), these groups had distinctive political motivations that accompanied their touted humanitarian ideals. Examining their origins and early motivations reveal characteristics that came to define these groups as activists within the fields of medicine and relief.

The Spanish Civil War and the AMBASD

> First of all there was an interest in Spain, a country trying, after years of repression, to be a democracy, and in a measure succeeding. So much I had read in newsprint. Then the Spanish government had sent a delegation to beg for American help, American sympathy. I went to a meeting. Yes, that was the beginning.[3]

Dr. Edward Barsky's words encapsulate the starting point for many of the Americans who became involved in sending medical aid to Spain. A native of New York, Barsky helped found the AMBASD and in January 1937 led the first volunteer unit of American doctors and nurses to Spain. The meeting he described took place in late October 1936 and featured two representatives of the Spanish Republican government. The difficulties they faced resonated with Barsky, who compared the Spanish struggle for democracy to America's own revolutionary history.

With reports of the rapidly deteriorating situation in Spain making their way across the Atlantic, Barsky became one of many U.S. citizens who felt compelled to respond to the crisis in ways that their government did not. By the end of the war, twenty-six organizations had registered with the U.S. State Department for licences to engage in relief activities to aid Republican Spain.[4] These organizations drew from a wide range of Americans, finding particular appeal among intellectuals, the political left, and certain immigrant and ethnic groups (including not only Spanish Americans, but African Americans and recent immigrants from Russia and Eastern Europe as well). Religious dimension also played a part, with Catholic groups in American generally being encouraged to support the Nationalists.[5] Meanwhile, influenced by the rise of fascism (and anti-Semitism) in central Europe, many Jewish Americans were drawn to support the Republican government, which came to represent an alternative to fascism. Supporting Spain's Second Republic became a sphere of action for Jewish Americans wishing to take a more proactive political stance against Nazi Germany, particularly with Germany's support of Spanish Nationalist forces.

Although dozens of aid organizations developed in support of the Spanish Republic, only a few assumed any real significance. The American Friends of Spanish Democracy (AFSD) was one of the first to appear. Led by Roger Baldwin, president of the American Civil Liberties Union, its mission was to raise public awareness about the Republican cause, collect donations for the Spanish Red Cross, and pressure the U.S. government to end the embargo.[6] The AFSD served as an umbrella organization for the creation of the American Medical Bureau and North American Committee. The activities of these subcommittees eventually eclipsed those of their founder and in January 1938 the American Medical Bureau and North American Committee formally combined forces to replace the AFSD as the American Medical Bureau and North American Committee to Aid Spanish Democracy.[7]

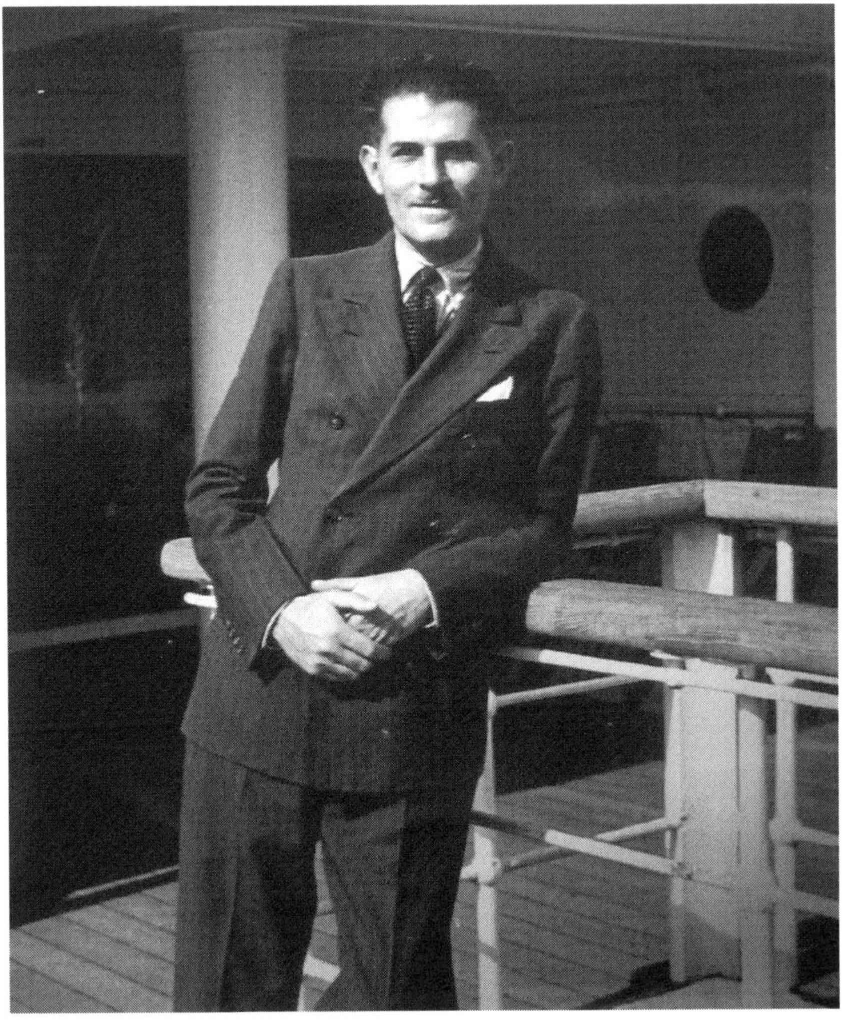

Figure 2. Edward Barsky en route to Spain. (Barsky Photograph Collection, Tamiment Library, New York University).

The Founders of the AMBASD

The physicians who helped establish the AMBASD were in many ways representative of the larger aid movement interested in Spain. A respected New York surgeon, Barsky was part of an informal group of physicians who met periodically to discuss contemporary affairs. Many of these men were colleagues at Beth Israel Hospital, where Barsky himself worked and which his father (also a physician) had helped found.[8] Other Beth Israel physicians present in the early discussions that led to the creation of the AMBASD were Dr. Irving Busch, Dr. Jesse Tomac, Dr. Benjamin Segal, and Dr. Milton Feltenstein.[9] A childhood friend of Barsky's, Busch later joined Barsky in Spain. Although Tomac, Segal, and Feltenstein never traveled to Spain themselves, they actively supported the organization from home throughout the war.

Even before the Spanish conflict, this group of physicians had demonstrated an interest in progressive causes and issues of international health. Several of those present had helped create Workers' Medical Aid, an organization established to provide medical care to strikers and their families along the New York waterfront.[10] Dr. Louis Miller had worked with the medical division of Herbert Hoover's American Relief Administration during the 1920s and was valued for his knowledge of the history of American medical relief abroad.[11] Others were experienced in the realities of military medicine. Colonel William J. Crookston had worked with the Red Cross during World War I and had served in the medical division of the U.S. armed forces in France.[12] All were well educated, with several—including Barsky—having completed part of their medical training in Europe. Like their colleagues who became involved in American aid to China, these individuals nurtured a sense of community that spanned both local and international spheres, and had already proven themselves committed to improving health within all levels of those communities.

Barsky traced the AMBASD's origins to a discussion held one October evening at Miller's house. With the Republican government reported as having practically no medical service of its own, the group reportedly began to discuss "American medical practice" as "never more needed."[13] The potential of American involvement followed as a matter of historical precedent. Other nationalities had already begun to act in support of the Republican cause. Dr. Feltenstein's wife, Evelyn Ahrend, an artist, had just returned from studying in France. While there, she witnessed the growing force of Republican sympathizers crossing the border into Spain, including the British Spanish Medical Aid Committee's first medical unit in early August.[14]

From New York to Nationwide

With these thoughts and convictions behind it, the AMBASD formally established itself as an affiliate of the AFSD on 21 October 1936. The AMBASD named Crookston as Executive Secretary and Miller as Chairman of the Executive Committee.[15] By the end of the month the AMBASD had established its main office in downtown New York City at 20 Vesey Street. Although the earliest discussions of the AMBASD's founders may have focused on the seemingly more achievable goals of simply fundraising to purchase ambulances and medical supplies, the goal of mounting a full medical "mission"—complete with personnel—was soon adopted.[16]

November and December were busy months. Collection boxes for donations were placed throughout Manhattan. A mass meeting at Madison Square Garden on 26 October 1936 attracted over 20,000 people and spurred the collection of almost $15,000.[17] As financial support flowed in for the project, the AMBASD expanded from its central New York hub. A national system of local and regional chapters developed—many of which were formed organically through local interest, only later to seek out affiliation with the New York based AMBASD for organizational and logistical support.[18] These developments were aided by the tour of a delegation of representatives of the Spanish government, which traveled across the country in December 1936 promoting the Republican cause.[19] By February 1937, branches of the AMBASD had been established in Philadelphia, Washington D.C., Baltimore, Boston, Buffalo, Toledo, Cleveland, Detroit, Grand Rapids, Chicago, San Francisco, and Miami.[20]

The AMBASD's national expansion was accompanied by an increasing number of public endorsements. By the end of the war, over half a dozen sub-committees of various professional groups supporting the AMBASD's activities had been established, with the support of various public figures. These included a Writers' and Artists' Committee, Social Workers' Committee, Musicians' Committee, Lawyers' Committee, Theatre Arts' Committee, Psychological Committee, and Women's Division.[21] Medical support came from the best universities and medical schools in the nation.[22] Dr. Henry Sigerist of Johns Hopkins University became an official sponsor of the AMBASD and was instrumental in organizing a Baltimore chapter. Dentist Dr. M.V. Loef did the same in Philadelphia, as did Stanford University's Dr. Thomas A. Addis in San Francisco. Harvard University's Dr. Walter B. Cannon, introduced earlier, helped with the establishment of a Boston Committee, before later assuming the position of national chairman.

As AMBASD founders sought to widen their base of support in the medical community, they found many of their supporters to be already established, like themselves, in sympathizing with and supporting liberal and progressive causes. A number of AMBASD medical committee members appear, for instance, in Eugene Perry Link's study of politically and socially progressive American physicians.[23] As Link argues, medicine and society were inextricably linked for physicians such as Cannon, Sigerist, and Sabin, who saw their professional role as carrying added responsibility in reinforcing positive social change. Not only that, but the physician's unique position in society gave him a particularly important role as an agent of change. While war may have been fundamentally "inimical to the ideals of the profession," and potentially a challenge to more socially minded physicians, it did not necessarily follow that such figures were pacifists. Sigerist, for example, made a point of differentiating between "the butchery of imperialist wars" and the more worthwhile "struggles to establish economic democracy."[24] Although violent conflict destroyed the physician's more immediate work toward health and wellness, it also presented an opportunity for greater and more far-reaching societal gains to be made. For progressive physicians such as Sigerist, the war in Spain was a natural fit for the latter.

The Volunteers

Gaining general support for their cause at home was one thing; finding volunteers willing to travel to the Spanish war zone to staff the AMBASD's projected hospitals and ambulance units was quite another. Volunteering to join the AMBASD meant leaving family and friends, and perhaps a job (which was often difficult to come by in the 1930s), to place oneself in the midst of an increasingly violent conflict thousands of miles away from home. Nevertheless, by the end of the war, almost 150 Americans had traveled to Spain as part of more than a dozen different AMBASD units. These volunteers included doctors, nurses, dentists, dental assistants, laboratory technicians, x-ray technicians, physical therapists, pharmacists, ambulance drivers and chauffeurs, engineers, cooks, and administrative assistants. While any attempt to provide a detailed biographical profile of this group as a whole is bound to be imperfect based on the limitations of available sources, some general patterns may still be discerned.[25]

Many AMBASD volunteers reported being drawn to the group through similar means. Public meetings and speaker events proved one of the most successful ways of attracting volunteers and support. Nurse Helen Freeman was one of those present at one of the group's first public meetings and later traveled to Spain with the first unit.[26] Late in 1937, nurse Ave Bruzzichesi heard Father O'Flanagan speak on behalf of the AMBASD and the Republican cause at the Hippodrome in New York City. Bruzzichesi was "so impressed by his speech and his appeal for volunteer medical aid" that she "immediately decided to go to Spain to offer what little aid [she] could as an individual."[27] Newspaper advertisements proved another way of finding volunteers. Dentist Dr. Zachary Stadt traced his involvement to a full-page advertisement he saw in the *New York Times*.[28] Nurse Sana Goldblatt also remembered a newspaper advertisement as having prompted her to apply to the AMBASD.[29] As their activities in Spain expanded, general news coverage of the AMBASD's activities also inspired support.[30]

The interest generated through word-of-mouth communication perhaps proved the most significant method of gathering recruits. Among a set of questionnaires completed by AMBASD volunteers decades later, nearly half of those who responded said that they had learned of the AMBASD through friends or professional colleagues.[31] In New York City, many were inspired by Barsky's example or encouraged directly by him to apply. Doctors and nurses from Beth Israel and other large urban hospitals (such as New York's Bellevue Hospital, Harlem Hospital, and Brooklyn Jewish Hospital) made a significant contribution to AMBASD units. As in the aid movement as a whole, New Yorkers showed particular interest in and dedication to the Republican cause.[32] Later on, San Francisco surgeon Dr. Leo Eloesser inspired a group of doctors and nurses to form their own Northern California unit. Promotion of the AMBASD by unions of nurses and hospital workers also helped recruitment efforts. As the first unit's head nurse Fredericka Martin later attested, "Someone from the nurses' union asked me if I would be willing . . . to leave my pleasant rut, and, of course, I was."[33] Nurse Ray Harris also remembered becoming involved through her union activities.[34]

Many prospective volunteers had demonstrated sympathy for progressive causes or political involvement in leftist, Socialist, or Communist groups. As historian Frances Patai concludes in her study of U.S. volunteer nurses in Spain, "these nurses were not inspired by romantic images of religion-motivated Florence Nightingale", but rather "were far more influenced by the early twentieth-century public health movement, concurrent new, radical, political ideas, and the Great Depression of the 1930s." Summarizing the demographics of the group based on her own research, Patai classifies most American nurses in Spain as products of a "new socio-political climate" in which nursing had become "a means for poor, immigrant and/or women of color to get satisfying, decent jobs and economic independence." Most were "urban poor or working-class children of immigrants from Eastern Europe or Russia" and more than half were secular Jews. While only 25 percent were Communist Party members by Patai's accounting, nearly all considered themselves liberals. Patai argues that volunteering for Spain became "an extension" of work they were already involved with in civil rights coalitions and union activities, all in response to the "collective disaster" of the Great Depression.[35]

Several of the volunteers who later joined AMBASD ranks traveled to Spain independently. Celia Greenspan followed her husband, a reporter for the *Daily Worker*, to Spain shortly after the outbreak of war.[36] Once there, she met the Canadian thoracic surgeon Dr. Norman Bethune. Bethune was setting up a mobile blood transfusion service for Republican Spain—the first service of its kind, relying on stored blood donations, and destined to become one of the primary medical innovations emerging from the war. Greenspan, trained as a laboratory technician, offered to help. After working with Bethune, she eventually moved on to the University Hospital in Murcia, where she became involved with the AMBASD, working as both a laboratory technician and nurse.[37]

Doctors Seymour Stanley Robbins and John L. Simon also traveled to Spain independently of the AMBASD. Both men worked directly under the auspices of the International Brigades as battalion doctors. Robbins, a cousin to one of Barsky's colleagues involved in the AMBASD's founding, had applied to go to Spain with the AMBASD, but was rejected for lack of sufficient experience.[38] Undaunted, Robbins decided to go on his own. Simon, too, had little medical experience when he went to Spain. Still a medical student, he volunteered with the International Brigades as a "first aid man," only later being promoted to the status of battalion doctor.[39] For medical students sympathetic to Republican Spain and wanting to become involved, the International Brigades offered a popular alternative. Hank Rubin was also still a student in medical school when the war broke out. He volunteered directly with the International Brigades, in which he served as both a soldier and a medic.[40] The examples of these men hint at the depth of motivation that drove so many (including medical volunteers) to go to Spain, as well as the selectivity shown by the AMBASD in choosing personnel. Dedication to the AMBASD's cause was important, but it was of limited use without the experience to back it up.

Another common entry into the AMBASD's medical forces was through the International Brigades. Wounded brigaders sometimes found their way into AMBASD units as ambulance drivers or mechanics. In the memoir of his experiences in Spain, ambulance driver James Neugass remembered two of such *chófers*:

> Marty & Bernie are each trained mechanics, truckdrivers and sterilizers. Marty is a twenty-seven-year-old ex-salesman of anti-freeze mixture from Philadelphia and Bernie, twenty-two, was a printer's apprentice back in New York. Both of them came to Spain through the international underground railway which sends voluntarios to fight in the International Brigades, and both had been transferred from the infantry into our front-line surgical unit because of their special technical skill.[41]

In this, the distinction between the volunteers of the AMBASD and those of the International Brigades becomes murkier—and such questions were important in the heated debates that developed both during the war and after.

AMBASD volunteers were subjected to a rigorous selection process. According to Barsky, as head of the personnel committee, the "right sort of people . . . must not be sentimentalists" and yet the AMBASD "could only take persons ready to die if necessary for their convictions."[42] Just as important was professional experience and "proven skill." For instance, "in the manner of chauffeurs," Barsky continued, "it meant nothing to us if a man could drive a car; he must also be an all round mechanic, perhaps an orderly, with the right stuff in him to make a nurse if necessary, and he must be young and healthy and mentally well-balanced."[43] Anticipating the challenges inherent to work in a war zone, those traveling to Spain needed to be reliable and able to cope with the difficulties they would face. This was even more important given their "volunteer" status: by their choice there was nothing officially requiring them to continue their work. Prospective volunteers had to submit a written application to be considered, followed by an interview and medical examination to confirm their interest, professional skill, and physical, and psychological capability.

In recalling the selection of personnel, Barsky commented in particular on the high number of "literary types" that came to the AMBASD offering their services, claiming talents and skills that were sometimes reported as going well beyond writing. Barsky attributed their presence to the AMBASD's "very impressive permit from the State Department licensing our work and permitting us to send personnel over-seas."[44] Under U.S. neutrality legislation, American citizens were not allowed to travel to Spain. The exception made for the AMBASD thus provided "a magic carpet" that such "literary gentlemen . . . were anxious to ride on." According to Barsky, these "men and women of imagination and more, of histrionic ability . . . came disguised as chauffeurs . . . as ambulance drivers, as mechanics, as male and female nurses and, I regret to say, sometimes as doctors."[45] The future of the AMBASD's special permission for travel to Spain, however, was not always certain as the U.S. State Department wavered in their official stance permitting medical volunteers to travel to a country otherwise off-limits to American citizens at the time. And for the vast majority of the AMBASD's medical volunteers, the motivations were deeper than Barsky's magic carpet ride for literary gentlemen.

One of these "literary types" (who developed a close working relationship with Barsky) was AMBASD ambulance driver James Neugass. Neugass became Barsky's personal driver, as well as a general ambulance driver. Despite Barsky's claimed skepticism of those with literary leanings, Neugass ultimately proved his dedication and skills as a driver. As Barsky later summarized in recommendation of Neugass's efforts, "Neugass has driven for me for the past five months, extremely loyal, willing and worked very hard. He drove at the front for four months under tremendous stress and danger and he also deserves every praise which he has rightly earned."[46] During his five months in Spain, Neugass kept a journal of his experiences. Returning to the U.S. in the spring of 1938 intending to convert his story into a book, Neugass died before his draft was ever published.[47]

Born to a wealthy Jewish family in New Orleans, Neugass spent much of the 1920s and 1930s bouncing between various universities, degrees, and odd jobs (which included teaching fencing and selling shoes), and traveling through Europe. As a union organizer and member of the Communist Party in the 1930s, Neugass joined the ranks of many Americans who opposed the rise of Hitler and Mussolini in Europe and saw the international movement of volunteers to Spain as an opportunity to fight back. But Neugass struggled with the motivations that brought him to Spain, even as he immersed himself in his work. Shortly after his arrival, Neugass wrote:

> I wish I knew more about war and about medicine. All I know is to drive, to take care of my car and to speak Spanish and to take orders . . . I'm certain that I don't like Franco and that I like democracy but I have seen nothing of fascism so far and much too much democracy. In my three weeks in Spain I believe I've learned that military strictness is necessary for the successful conduct of any war, that elections during wartime seem a little absurd and that the degree of discipline necessary to win the war counterfeits what many people might think was fascism.[48]

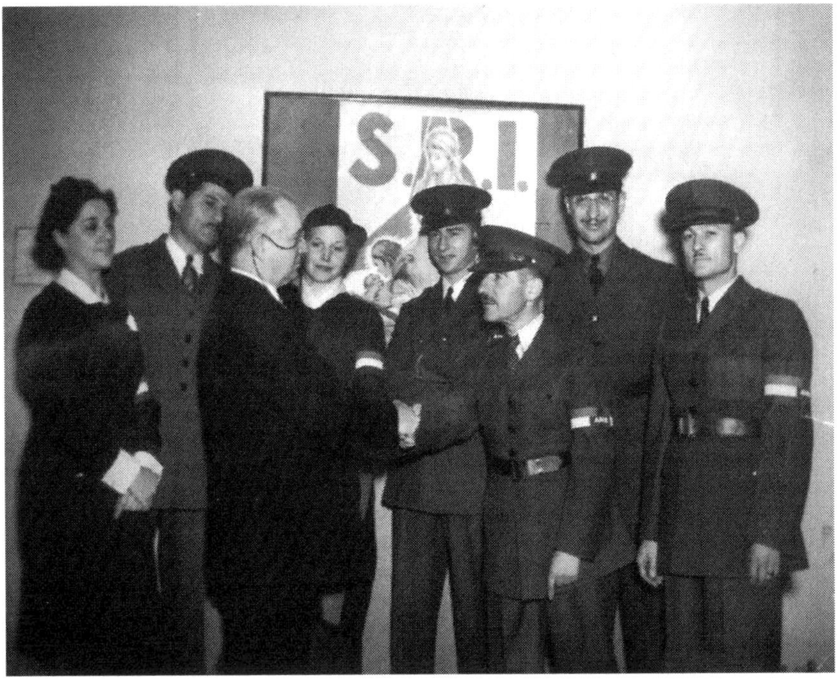

Figure 3. Barsky (second from left) and Neugass (second from right) prepare for departure with a group of AMBASD volunteers, including Nurse Ave Bruzzichesi (far left) and Dr. Leo Eloesser (front right, shaking hands). (Barsky Photograph Collection, Tamiment Library, New York).

Neugass's political views were clearly an important part of his decision to travel to Spain. In fact, Neugass claimed, if it were not for his poor eyesight, he might have volunteered for the infantry. As much as Hemingway and others may have made the ambulance driver/writer into a heroic figure, Neugass also opposed it. In his own words, he described himself as "still ashamed of driving an ambulance," disliking the "literary, intellectual, here-to-be-revolted-by-the-horror-of-war, later-to-write-a-book, Allan Seager mock heroism tradition that lies behind my job."[49] His frustration became even more pronounced as he waited for orders to leave for the front. Simply being in Spain was not enough—part of him described wishing to be tested by fire. Seeing so many wounded gave Neugass a sense of inferiority for not committing enough to the cause he supported. Neugass's motivations for going to Spain were complex. While his memoir provides and exceptional account in the detail of one person's story, it also offers clues to the other factors that instigated AMBASD volunteer involvement.

The Motivations

The conditions of the decade's economic depression became motivations in and of themselves for many volunteers. American society was in social, political, and economic upheaval. As Dr. Albert Byrne observed simply in describing his own motivations in going to Spain, Spain offered an opportunity to "at last be useful" in a time when "M.Ds [sic] seemed to be the most redundant things on the market."[50] Before going to Spain, Byrne had worked as a doctor at a series of transient camps established as a New Deal program in New Jersey. When these were shut down, he moved back to New York, where he joined the staff at Bellevue Hospital. It was there—through his peripheral involvement in the hospital workers' union—he first heard about Spain. Similarly, dentist Jack Klein attributed his decision to go to Spain both to political sympathies and his "inability to establish a firm base" either "professionally or economically."[51] Meanwhile, physical therapist Eugenia Grunsky noted frankly that while humanitarian motives could have played a part, more important was that she needed work, even "escape" from her life at home. Although she "knew vaguely [she] was against Hitler and Mussolini and Franco" it was "certainly not" any political awareness that drove her to Spain.[52] However, Grunsky seems to have been more the exception than the rule.

For many volunteers, humanitarian and political motivations for going to Spain were not necessarily distinguishable. In a questionnaire circulated among surviving AMBASD veterans several decades after the war, most respondents cited having been motivated to volunteer for both political and humanitarian reasons.[53] Most political orientations were reported as broadly anti-Fascist. As laboratory technician Dorothy Fontaine remembered, "I was naïve enough to believe that Fascism, if stopped in Republican Spain, might prevent a second world war!"[54]

When nurse Irene Goldin was asked why she wanted to go to Spain, she reportedly replied, "to fight against fascism."[55] For many volunteers, Spain marked a turning point in their political awareness—or "loss of political innocence," as put by laboratory technician Morris Kornblum—as vague political leanings were transformed into more definite ideas.[56] Most, it seems, saw their interest in aiding the people of Republican Spain as a basic humanitarian impulse that was a fundamental part of their broader ideology. It was not a choice between being political and being humanitarian—the humanitarian interests they described were integral to their developing political views.

In contrast with many of their counterparts at work in China, the majority of those involved in the AMBASD did not have direct ties to Spain before

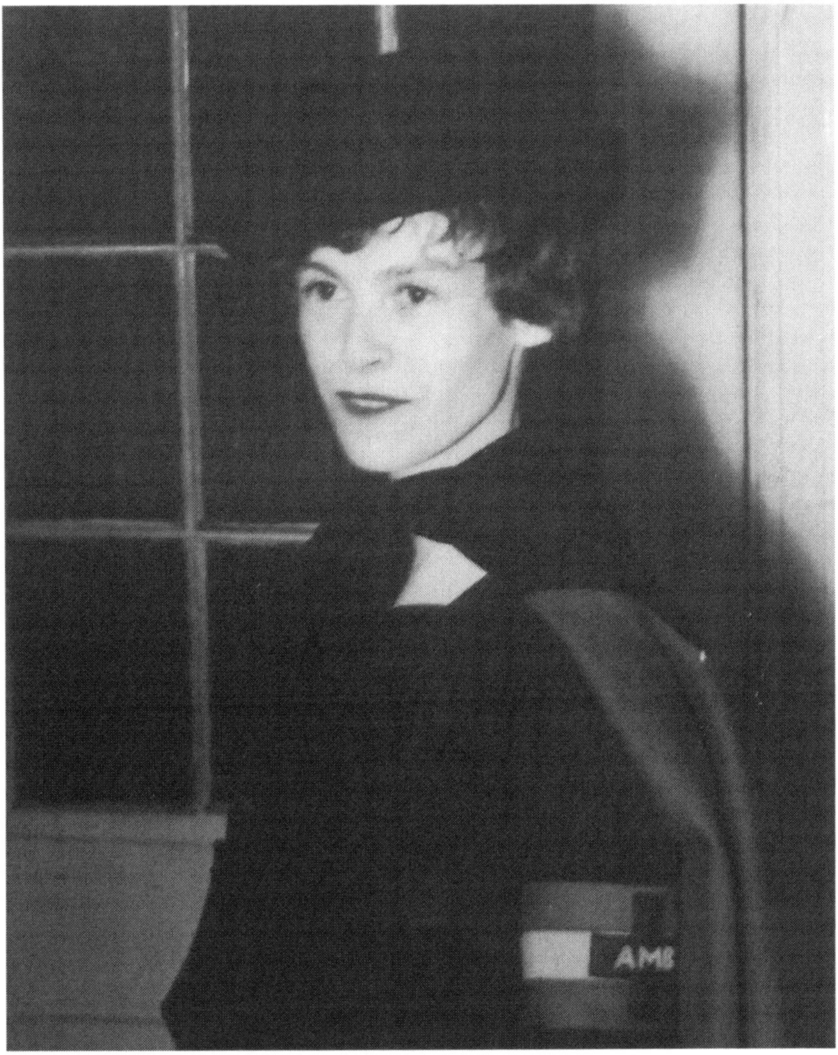

Figure 4. Laboratory technician Dorothy (Dotty) Fontaine (Martin Photograph Collection, Tamiment Library, New York).

volunteering. Certainly the historical relationship between Spain and the U.S. was not that of China and the U.S. in terms of immigration history. Connections between the U.S. and Spain, as expressed in the development of the AMBASD, seem more illustrative of their common Western and European cultural heritage. If the AMBASD found greater support among any ethnic or religious group, it was among Jewish-Americans, many of who had emigrated (or had family who emigrated) from central or Eastern Europe. For these individuals, interest in Spain stemmed from an awareness of the rise of Fascism in Europe—and concern for the implications that would have not only in Europe, but in the U.S. as well. Meanwhile, Americans with personal ties to China saw a similarly alarming sequence of events underway in Asia.

The Rockefeller Foundation also had its own traditions of work in both Spain and China, although its activities in China have been perhaps more significant.[57] Beginning in the 1920s, the Rockefeller Foundation's International Health Board sent a series of experts to help assess Spain's public health needs and offer support to developing a stronger system. The Rockefeller Foundation offered funding to indigenous efforts against malaria and ankylostomiasis, helped support the renovation of regional health centres in Cáceras, Albacete, and Vallecas, and provided a fellowship scheme enabling over three dozen Spanish doctors and nurses to gain expertise in public health through studies in the United States.[58] None of these efforts, however, sought to develop entirely new systems, but rather (at the request of Spanish health authorities) offered financial support to renovate existing infrastructure.[59]

The Second Sino-Japanese War and the ABMAC

By the time the first unit of volunteers arrived in Spain, war was well underway in China. And what Dr. Barsky was for American medical relief to Republican Spain, Dr. Frank Co Tui became for American medical aid to Nationalist China.

Co Tui had been born in Amoy (Xiamen) China in 1897, but moved to the Philippines with his parents when he was nine years old. He called the Philippines home for the next seventeen years, during which time he earned both his A.B. (1917) and M.D. (1922) from the University of the Philippines. In 1923, Co Tui moved to the United States with his Philippine wife, Praxedes Tanda. By 1937, he had established a professional life in New York City, having served on the faculty of New York University's School of Medicine for three years as a professor of experimental surgery.[60] Remembered by friends as a modest and humble man, Co Tui evoked the memory in one friend of "an Asian Igor Stravinsky, gnome-like, spare but with the same jaunty walk . . . or of a smaller edition of the fictional Ichabod Crane."[61] Remembered by others for his "fiery" personality, Co Tui became a fierce proponent of the ABMAC's work and played a critical role in the organization's early development.[62] Serving as vice president of the organization, in addition to chairing the group's Needs and Disbursements Committee, Co Tui played a particularly important role in building up the group's connections with prominent individuals and organizations in Nationalist China. In 1942 the Nationalist government awarded him the Order of the Brilliant Jade for his service.[63] After the war, Co Tui returned to the Philippines, where he continued to work as a physician until his death in 1983.

Alongside Dr. Co Tui in the ABMAC's roster of founding members were Dr. Farn B. Chu and Mr. Joseph Wei. Dr. Farn B. Chu was a second-generation

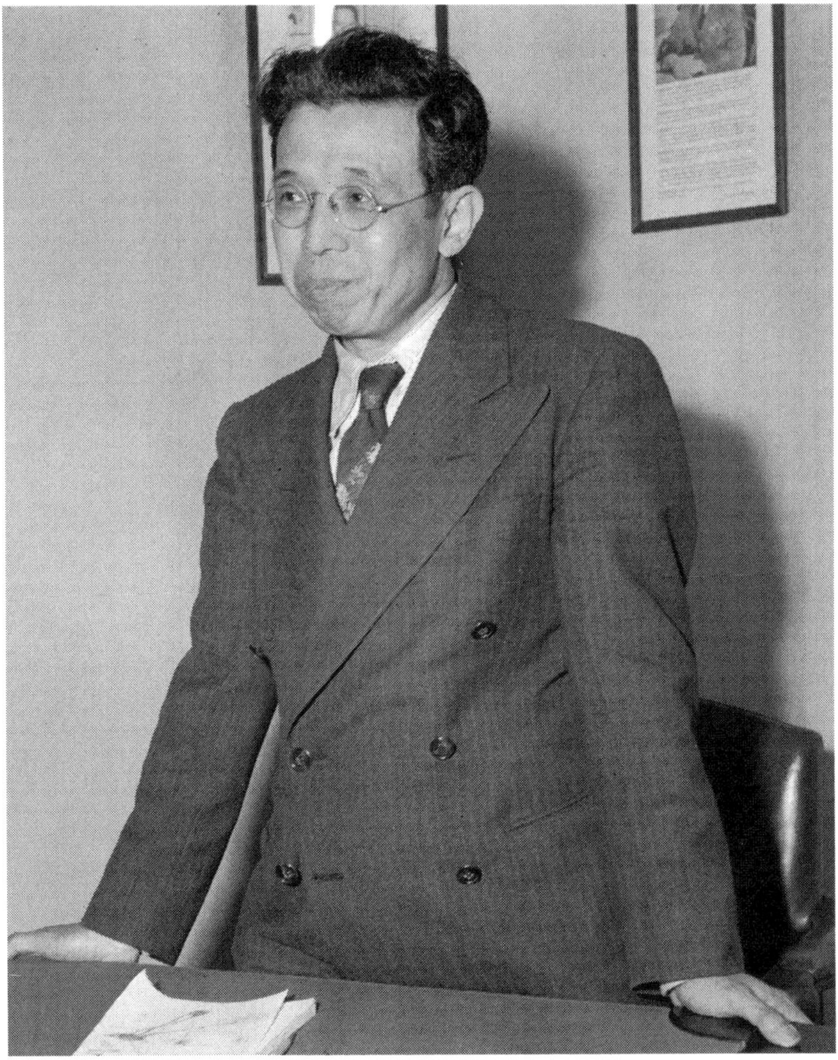

Figure 5. Dr. Frank Co Tui (ABMAC Records, Rare Book and Manuscript Library, Columbia University).

Chinese-American, born in New York City in 1906. Coming from a large family, with four brothers and three sisters, Chu completed his undergraduate degree at Columbia University in 1926 before going on to receive his M.D. from Yale Medical School in 1930. Chu returned to the New York area after graduation, completing his internship at Jersey City General Hospital and at Morrisania Hospital (in the Bronx). Chu continued to practice in the Bronx and in Manhattan's upper east side (at Lenox Hill Hospital and the Hospital for the Ruptured and Crippled) until his death in 1941. His obituary described him as "a widely known member of the Chinese community" who "preferred to live among his own people, although he had as many American as Chinese patients."[64] Dr. Chu's wife, who was from Shanghai, played an equally active role in the ABMAC's early years, helping organize a popular series of banquet-style dinners in Chinatown to raise money for the organization.[65]

Like Co Tui, the ABMAC's third founder, Mr. Joseph Wei, was a more recent addition to New York City. Born in Shanghai in 1902 to a Chinese pharmacist, Wei was a professional outlier in the trio of ABMAC founders, pursuing business rather than medicine. Wei's early education, however, lay in engineering and political activism. Growing up amid the political turbulence following the Chinese revolution in 1911, Wei showed an early interest in Chinese politics. At seventeen, Wei helped lead demonstrations against China's signing of the Versailles Treaty when the Allies refused to incorporate guarantees of Chinese territoriality. In the early 1920s, Wei traveled to the U.S. to continue his studies in Engineering. After completing his B.A. at Purdue University, Wei returned to China to work, although would again return to the U.S. in 1935 to manage the American affiliate of a Chinese trading organization. When Wei received recognition from the Chinese government for his services with the Order of the Brilliant Jade, he commented that he was "grateful" for the award, but "embarrassed . . . as it should be a Chinese citizen's duty to do his utmost."[66] Although resident in the U.S., Wei's involvement in the ABMAC stemmed from his personal ties and sense of civic obligation to his home country. Eventually, in 1943, after "considerable frustration as an alien," Wei "was admitted into the Baldwin Locomotive Works in Eddystone, PA, as an inspector of tank and gun parts, engines, and locomotives."[67] Wei continued to serve on the ABMAC Board of Directors well into the 1980s.

The ABMAC first arose one October evening in 1937 when these three friends—Co Tui, Chu, and Wei—and their wives met for dinner in New

York City. Discussing the latest events in China, they discussed the possibility of starting an organization to address Chinese medical needs. Before long, the idea gained momentum and, with the support of the Chinese consul general, Dr. Tsune-Chi Yü, the ABMAC was christened with the motto "Humanity Above All."[68] The ABMAC thus framed its initial inception within the noble language of neutral humanitarian aid, unpolluted by political ideology. However, in clearly defining the intended recipients of its efforts in national terms, the group simultaneously painted itself in a more political light.

Although borrowing strikingly similar language in name to the AMBASD, the leaders of the ABMAC sought to distance themselves from their Spanish counterparts early on. Shortly after the war broke out in China, Dr. Walter B. Cannon made a public announcement offering the AMBASD's Fourth Avenue Headquarters in New York City to colleagues aiding the Chinese. "To all friends of China," Cannon was quoted, "the Medical Bureau [to Aid Spanish Democracy] offers the services of the noted medical men who compose our national advisory board. It offers the services of our technical staff, which has gained experience in establishing American hospitals in Spain and maintaining a staff of 113 doctors, nurses and ambulance drivers."[69] Although Cannon himself later became involved in campaigns for China through both the New England Committee for China Relief and later the ABMAC, the ABMAC showed little interest in Cannon's offer on behalf of the AMBASD. As observed bluntly by Co Tui in 1939, "To have China's cause identified with leftism in the eyes of America would be suicidal" and would "do for China what was done for Spain: raise a total of two and one half millions among liberals but to hopelessly prejudice the cause."[70] In this quote, Co Tui's comments appear less a reflection of his personal political views than a calculated analysis of the dominant American political and social culture—and, ultimately, the society whose support was sought.

Despite Co Tui's hesitance to risk any affiliation with Spanish aid efforts, the ABMAC's first weeks and months of activities appear remarkably similar to those of the AMBASD. The ABMAC began its fundraising efforts directly soliciting funds through mailings and street campaigns. As New York City shoppers bustled about the city for holiday shopping, "over 100 Chinese high school and college students solicited funds from passersby . . . as each waved in one hand a wood standard bearing a placard and in the other shook a duly licensed metal can."[71] By November 1937 over $8,000 had been raised, which went toward the purchase of tetanus antitoxin, chloroform, bandages, and ambulances to send to China.[72]

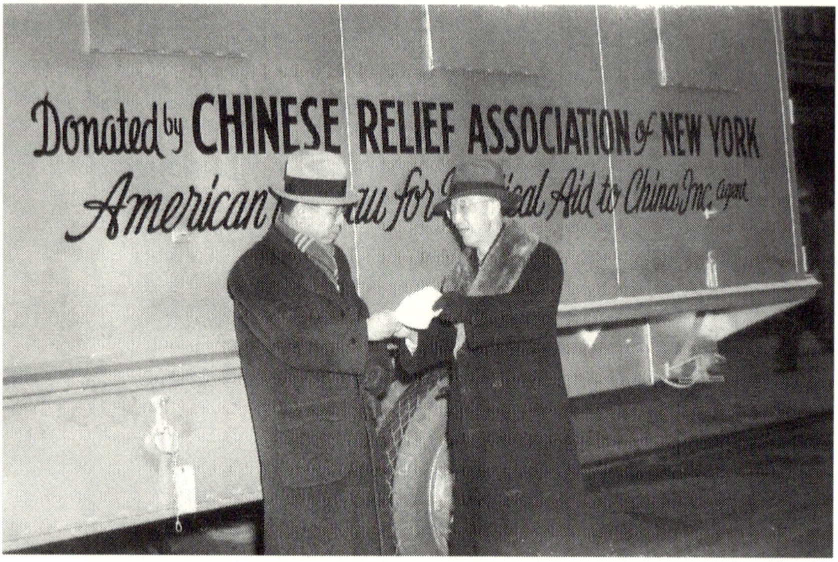

Figure 6. Co Tui (left) at a fundraising event in New York City's Chinatown (ABMAC Records, Rare Book and Manuscript Library, Columbia University).

From this foundation, a steady expansion followed. By the end of January 1938, the ABMAC was incorporated under New York corporation law and set its next goal at $35,000, which it hoped to raise in cooperation with the United Council for Civilian Relief in China.[73] By the end of February, the ABMAC had expanded nationwide into a network of local and regional chapters from its base in New York City. San Francisco, with its large Chinese-American population, became another important center for activity, although New York City remained the central hub. By June 1938, donations had funded eight hundred thousand doses of cholera vaccine and six ambulance chassis, with a dedicated $1,000 for the Hankow Rest house and $1,000 for the University Hospital in Nanking.[74] In July, the ABMAC negotiated an agreement with an American pharmaceutical company, which promised to donate $1,000 a week for six months.[75]

Meanwhile, the ABMAC continued to raise money through the cultural sphere in a series of fundraising dinners and other events. The group helped organize the visit of a Chinese theatrical group, whose tour of "An Evening in Cathay" raised $2,000. That same year marked the beginning of the Bowl of Rice parties—inspired by the Chinese saying that "a bowl of rice is worth a thousand gold pieces"—in which guests bought tickets to a Chinese meal centred around a bowl of rice.[76] The San Francisco chapter, which broke organization records for fundraising with the leadership of Paul C. Smith (managing editor for the San Francisco Chronicle), raised $48,000 in 1938.[77]

Especially early in the campaign, communities of Chinese Americans provided crucial support. In Co Tui's own words, the "stunned inactivity of the American public" immediately following the Japanese invasion of China "was succeeded in some quarters by a profound defeatism engendered by the enormity of the relief task," while in others "the neutrality-in-all-things attitude prevailed," and with "progressives . . . preoccupied with Spain and other European crises . . . the result was that while the Chinese communities poured forth their money, the response from the American public was very meagre."[78] Particularly given their long history of unequal treatment in the United States, supporting China became an important political expression for many Chinese Americans.[79] When Sun Yat-sen, revolutionary and founder of the Chinese Nationalist Party, traveled to Hawaii to recruit support for his anti-Manchu ideas, he found a wellspring of popular support among politically disenfranchised Chinese-Americans who had been excluded from many aspects of American life.[80] When Sun Yat-sen's revolutionary ideas carried the day in the Chinese Revolution of 1911, Chinese-Americans reportedly rejoiced.

In the decades that followed, however, China's internal political situation deteriorated as feuds between national powers and regional warlords drove the country into civil war. When China's Nationalist Party reorganized Chinese politics as a unifying force for a range of patriotic movements, it simultaneously offered a cohesive political unit around which Chinese living abroad could rally. Japan's incursion into China's Shandong Province in 1928 both established a common enemy and inspired the creation of anti-Japanese groups such as the Chinese Citizens' Patriotic League of New York. When full-scale war broke out less than a decade later, in 1937, such organized forms of support for China gained an even stronger foothold in the United States.

That same year, an emergency meeting between ninety-one Chinese American organizations in San Francisco established the Chinese War Relief Association of America. Aiming to provide overseas assistance to the Nationalist government, the China War Relief Association raised money, organized demonstrations, promoted a boycott of Japanese goods, and picketed shipyards in California, Washington, and Oregon to prevent the shipment of scrap iron—and other possible war materiel—to Japan.[81] Miscevic and Kwong's classification of such organized political activities by Chinese Americans as "People's Diplomacy" suggests a valuable historical framework for understanding the establishment and development of the ABMAC.[82] But the leaders of the ABMAC sought more than popular support. As Co Tui wrote, "American civilization is strictly a business civilization and business interests have a larger factor in determining action than sentimental ones, specially [sic] now-a-days—with a depression and ten million unemployed. But if humanitarian interests and business interests can be made to coincide then the result will be doubly effective."[83]

Rockefeller Medicine and the Missionary Legacy

Although not directly operating from the business realm, the philanthropic arm of John D. Rockefeller's industrial wealth also had a significant history of influence in China. Shortly after its expansion into the international arena with the establishment of the International Health Board in 1913, the Rockefeller Foundation formed a separate division dedicated to promoting Western medicine in China. Within a year of its founding in 1914, the China Medical Board (CMB) planned to establish two medical schools in China. Although only one of these eventually became a reality, the Peking Union Medical College (PUMC) became a major force in Chinese medical education. As observed by a member of UCR stationed in China, "I have been struck time and again by the fact that although the PUMC graduated very few students, medicine in China today seems to be run pretty much by its graduates."[84]

ABMAC founders recruited early support from a number of former PUMC faculty in the U.S., many of whom were also outstanding figures in New York City's community of academic medicine. Dr. Frank Meleney and Dr. Donald D. Van Slyke were two such recruits. Meleney became second vice president of the ABMAC in February 1938, and was later given credit for recruiting Dr. George Vincent—former president of the Rockefeller Foundation and the University of Minnesota—to the ABMAC presidency in May 1938.[85] Meleney and Van Slyke offered the ABMAC access to the PUMC's American-based fundraising organization, the Yü Wang Fu Association. Both Meleney and Van Slyke were professors at Columbia's College of Physicians & Surgeons. Other faculty, including former associate dean Dr. Aura Severinghaus, plastic surgeon Dr. Jerome Webster, physiologist Dr. Magnus Gregerson, and surgeon Dr. George H. Humphreys II, all played important roles in ABMAC development.[86]

As evidenced by a glimpse into the faculty networks described above, formal academic exchange between China and the U.S. also contributed to the construction of networks of aid. Such exchanges had a substantial history, started under U.S. presidents Theodore Roosevelt and William Howard Taft, and later expanded with the Boxer Indemnity Scholarship Program.[87] Many private American universities also established satellite programs in China during the first decades of the twentieth century.[88] The establishment of such soft power approaches offered a foundation for later diplomatic claims made by the ABMAC and UCR for the potential of emergency relief and investment in Chinese healthcare infrastructure and medical education to have a wider impact.

As educational exchanges sought to translate American and Chinese cultural experiences, American missionary groups had an even longer history in both exporting American culture and ideals abroad and interpreting and promoting Chinese culture to American audiences. As Dean Acheson (later secretary of state under President Harry S. Truman) once commented, "Hardly a town in our land was without its society to collect funds and clothing for Chinese missions, to worry about those who labored in distant, dangerous and exotic vineyards of the Lord, and to hear the missionaries 'inspiring reports.'"[89] The first two decades of the twentieth century, in particular, had been a "golden age" for American missionaries in China, although the movement faced a challenge from the simultaneous rise of Chinese nationalism, which often targeted American missionaries as dangerous allies of other imperial economic and political intrusions into Chinese sovereignty and self-determination. Partially in response to such criticisms, evangelists of the social gospel, who put greater emphasis on improving conditions of poverty, ill health, and educational inequalities, rose in prominence. As a movement within the American Protestant missionary community, proponents of the social gospel argued for the importance of going beyond the focus on individual salvation to address the basic social needs of the communities they served.[90] In many ways, this shift in priorities became a natural precursor to more secular aid efforts.

Walter Judd offers a dynamic example of someone who transitioned between missionary work in China to more secular (and political) avenues of involvement. Growing up amid a large family in small-town Nebraska, Judd worked his way through his undergraduate and medical training at the University of Nebraska. After serving with the U.S. Army in World War I, Judd earned his medical degree in 1923. Active with the Student Volunteer Movement (a missionary service organization founded by university students in 1886), Judd first traveled to China in 1926, sponsored by the Congregational Foreign Missionary Board.[91] During his time in China, Judd had counted himself among the new wave of missionaries, critiquing predecessors for remaining isolated within a "miniature home land" or "little America," in which they indulged overriding loyalties to "their own blood, language, flag, and culture."[92] In many ways, this criticism would find later echoes in attitudes among the ABMAC toward the "Old China Hands." In reference to the missionaries and businessmen that had once been seen as the dominant modes of cultural exchange between the U.S. and China, the term was used as a catchall for older attitudes of "paternal, even colonial" control of Chinese enterprise. By the estimation of ABMAC leaders, "Old China Hands" had become "the main interpreters of the Chinese people in America," while rarely coming "into intimate contact with Chinese life and culture."[93]

When Judd returned to the U.S. in 1938, his experience in China helped to fuel the development of his political career. Judd had become a prominent supporter of Chiang Kai-shek—giving 1,400 speeches in forty-six states over two years on behalf of the American Committee for Non-Participation in Japanese Aggression.[94] Seeking to alert Americans to the threat of Japanese aggression, Judd urged a boycott of Japanese goods and a halt to the supply of war materiel from the U.S. government well before Pearl Harbor, his interests turned increasingly toward politics. In 1943 he was elected Republican representative to the U.S. Congress, kicking off a twenty-year political career.[95] While Judd's sustained interest in promoting an internationalist vision of America's place in world affairs linked him with collaborators from both sides of the political aisle (Judd and Democratic senator Harry S. Truman spent two weeks in 1943 traveling around the U.S. to promote the United Nations), his stringent anti-Communism kept him in close alliance with right-wing groups.[96] In the years leading up to World War II, Judd's activism helped to build support for the ABMAC as well. Sharing his observations of the products of Japanese aggression at one of the group's early gatherings, Judd offered unequivocal and vivid reports of the brutality and atrocities committed by Japanese forces.[97] Drawn by his experience in China as a medical missionary, Judd's presence in the ABMAC highlights another important dimension of the ABMAC's earliest American support.[98]

While both educational exchange and missionary work prepared many for support of the ABMAC, there were always exceptions, of which Dr. Maurice William was one. Dr. William, the ABMAC's first secretary and member of the board of directors, was a dentist with clearly defined political ideas. As a young man working a series of menial jobs, William became heavily involved in the Socialist movement. Having emigrated to the U.S. from Russia with his family when he was eight years old, William sought his first professional degree in law. However, he dropped out of his part-time course after hearing New York City Socialist congressman Meyer London denounce the profession as "parasitic."[99] Searching for a new career path that would take him beyond delivering newspapers and working twelve hours a day in a dairy shop, William settled on dentistry, completing his degree in 1907. Observing the daily struggles of working-class New Yorkers—accompanied by a sense of disillusionment following World War I—eventually led William to reassess the Marxist ideas he had previously espoused. Highly critical of the standards of care practiced in these lower-income settings for dental care, William became a vocal advocate for legislation to improve New York standards of care for practicing dentists. In 1920, he articulated his own larger philosophy in the self-published book, *The Social Interpretation of History.*

Analyses of Chinese revolutionary (and physician) Sun Yat-sen's writing suggest that William's *Social Interpretation* had a powerful impact far beyond U.S. borders. As pointed out by University of Chicago historian Harley Farnsworth MacNair in 1930, "In paragraph after paragraph, Dr. Sun either quoted, almost word for word, or paraphrased, the arguments which he had found in the Social Interpretation of History. He now repudiated several of his own earlier theories, substituting therefore the system of thought which he had recently discovered in Dr. William's work."[100] In deviating from the Marxist philosophy he had previously espoused, William turned from a focus on the industrial proletariat to the consumer as the driving force of history. William's experience as a dentist serving New York's poor informed the development of his own social ideas. Building on his professional interest in improving health on an individual basis, William increasingly turned his attention to improving the health of society as a whole.

Despite its conscious efforts to avoid leftist affiliations, the ABMAC eventually found itself in a loose alliance with the left-wing CAC. Like the ABMAC, the CAC also established itself in New York City in the fall of 1937 with the aim of providing material medical relief to China. However, the CAC chose to focus on sending this aid to China's Northwest provinces, where the Chinese Communists maintained control. Although associated most directly with Chinese Communist forces through Madame Sun Yat-sen's China Defence League, the CAC also worked with Dr. Robert Lim of the Chinese Red Cross, alongside the ABMAC.

Unfortunately, the profiles of those behind the CAC's foundation in the U.S. remain murky. Before joining the larger organization of United China

Relief, there are very few historical references to the CAC's activities. As of August 1938 (roughly a year after its initial founding), a man named Oliver Haskell had taken on CAC leadership as director.[101] Haskell had first traveled to China as a student in 1929 with the Pomona College Oriental Expedition—a year-long trip taken by ten students from Pomona College in Los Angeles, California.[102] Like so many other Americans (including those involved in the ABMAC), Haskell's interest in China arose out of an educational exchange sponsored by private American institutions of higher education.[103]

Before joining the CAC, Haskell had worked in organizing textile workers for the Congress of Industrial Organizations. Haskell's main work for the CAC seemed to involve traveling the U.S. speaking on behalf of the organization. Recalling a conference in San Francisco's Chinatown for Chinese benevolent organizations, Haskell described Chinese-American support dominating the scene of aid, just as Co Tui and the ABMAC had reported. However, Haskell painted a slightly more negative portrait of such donations:

> The problem they had was raising money from the American public for China aid. They were bleeding the Chinese community. Really bleeding them. They would march a Chinese merchant into the shrine in the back of the Chinese six companies in San Francisco, make him kneel down in front of this shrine and swear on the bones of his ancestors that he was giving all he could. They would know what his balance sheet was and they would tell him how much was enough. But they could not get any money from the American public because they didn't know how. They weren't organized to do that. So I spoke about the techniques that could be used by the Chinese, in Duluth or Tacoma or wherever they were, to get money from the American public for China aid.

Even at these meetings, amid crowds predisposed to aiding China, Haskell's political orientation became a source of controversy. As he remembered later, it was his three-year involvement in the CAC that "got the Un-American Committee most excited" when he worked for the Los Angeles Housing Authority.[104]

Intersections of Activism and Medicine

Although the ABMAC and the CAC operated within different political spheres in China and the U.S., both drew from the model of medical activism described in this study. With the personal interests of their earliest supporters drawing from networks of missionary work and educational exchange between China and the U.S., the leadership of the ABMAC and the CAC sought to simultaneously express political sympathies and humanitarian ideals through professional expertise. They became both interpreters of Chinese history and culture for Americans at home, and exporters of American ideals abroad. In this sense, the ABMAC and the CAC became a new mode of cultural exchange. Just as the "secular journalists" had become "the new publicists for American images of China and the Chinese," the ABMAC and the CAC picked up a similar tradition of the social gospel in the secular terms of the Western medical tradition.[105] The medical activists of the ABMAC and the CAC sought to exercise a political voice, mediated through medicine. As argued in the ABMAC's own historical account, "ABMAC's continuous and expanding activity . . . kept the American people constantly posted on Japanese aggression in China, and undoubtedly contributed toward the development of a more favorable attitude to China."[106]

Considering past historical reviews of American contacts with China in the decades leading up to the outbreak of the war, what is perhaps most striking in all is the general sympathy such outgoing individuals ended up feeling with the communities that they entered—whether Communist or Nationalist, religious or secular. Regardless of their purpose, they reported more similarities than differences with the people they met. As noted by Shewmaker in his survey of American interactions with Chinese Communism from 1927 to 1945, "whatever their background, [Americans] almost invariably returned from Yenan aglow with praise for China's Communists."[107] And certainly those of ABMAC seeking to bolster the Nationalist cause seemed to show equal respect for their counterparts. Whether they sympathized with Nationalists or Communists, Americans consistently seemed to read their own culture and priorities into those they supported.

And yet, the people of the ABMAC and CAC differentiated themselves from the broader American populace by their dedication to the cause of China as fuelled by such perceptions. But considering the fact that most had other avenues of engagement with Chinese people and institutions, what was it about the ABMAC that triggered their involvement? In 1937, the Rockefeller Foundation's China Medical Board was still actively supporting medical work through the PUMC. And medical missionaries—although decreased in number—were still active through clinics and medical schools associated with American missions. Private American universities still operated campuses overseas. Meanwhile, several independent physicians and nurses had proven that one didn't have to belong to a pre-existing institutional network to immerse oneself in medical work in China. What did the ABMAC or the CAC offer that was different from these other options? Why did their supporters feel the need to start a new program, outside of the avenues of cultural and medical engagement in China that had first introduced them to the country?

First, these new private organizations were based on forming a response to the urgent medical needs created by violent conflict, which contrasted sharply with the educational orientation of established infrastructure connecting medical communities in the U.S. and China. From its earliest days, the Rockefeller Foundation had sought to differentiate its philanthropic activities from those of charitable relief by emphasizing long-term investments in infrastructure or simpler transfers of money or supplies. The China Medical Board and PUMC remained true to this mission, even amid the escalation of war. The PUMC continued its activities more or less uninterrupted until the Japanese temporarily took over the school in their occupation of Peking. But the perceived lack of engagement in the war effort also brought criticism against the PUMC. According to Claude Forkner of the China Medical Board and representative of the Rockefeller Foundation during the war years, "PUMC grads had become too Americanized, over-isolated from social conditions," and "unable to adapt to problem situations."[108] Meanwhile, mission- and university-sponsored medical schools emphasized parallel orientations directed toward long-term investment in education based on the American institutional model.

Secondly, in building out of a response to war, the majority of those involved in the new private medical relief organizations discussed had secondary political motivations that served as an added impetus for their involvement. As noted by Dr. Robert R. Williams in describing his own motivations for becoming an ABMAC director in the early 1940s, "My main interests have always been democracy and medicine, and I feel that my interest in the former is due chiefly to my residence in the East. I am delighted therefore to join . . . in a work which combines my interest in democracy and in medicine and health."[109]

Conclusions

The negotiation of response to foreign conflict constitutes one of the central practices of international relations, with opinion often revolving around the central issues of the role of war in society and the potential of violence or non-violence to mediate a peace. The Spanish Civil War and the Second Sino-Japanese War were no exception. Arising in the period between the two world wars, these more localized conflicts presented a sharp dilemma to aspirations to keep a global peace. In the U.S., though physically isolated from such distant violence, Americans found their sympathies piqued, for a variety of reasons. Armed with personal, political, and professional rationales, U.S. citizens began to coalesce into groups seeking to take action abroad, where they saw more established systems failing to act.

The complex combination of personal, political, and professional motivations behind private aid efforts in the U.S. were not new. The inherent challenges to so-called "neutral" aid have a long history across a diverse range of conflicts and circumstances. From what is left of their voices in the historical record, it seems that few, if any, of those individuals behind the AMBASD, ABMAC, or CAC would have described their personal involvement in foreign aid efforts as entirely neutral in intent. But perhaps their efforts may have been hoped to be neutralizing in their impact: seeing perceived injustices abroad, their efforts sought to counteract those forces. While these groups claimed to be exceptional compared to the status quo in their approach and action, they also built consciously upon prior waves of U.S. humanitarian activism abroad. In so doing, the American Red Cross became a prime example—and subject of critique. And yet its parallels with the new private aid efforts of the late 1930s are significant, particularly in the targeted relationships between private aid and military medical services. In some ways, the AMBASD, ABMAC, and CAC provide a model of how political and professional activism was translated into organizational change. How did these groups respond to and define themselves in light of their predecessors?

CHAPTER TWO

Institutional Failure
Replacing the Red Cross?

As the leader in private aid in times of war, the story of the Red Cross—in both its national and international forms—provides both a parallel and a contrast to the development of the AMBASD, ABMAC, and CAC. On the one hand, as private responses to conflict growing out of a basic critique of existing services available to the wounded and the victims of war, there are commonalities between the private aid organizations of this study and the International Committee of the Red Cross (ICRC) and affiliated national societies such as the American Red Cross (ARC). On the other hand, by the late 1930s, the ICRC and ARC were not the same organizations they had been at their founding. Since World War I, the Red Cross had become the dominant figure in international medical relief in times of war. With the expansion of Red Cross activities and services, however, the military medical services of the nations involved in World War I had also established new standards. As noted briefly in an ARC memorandum prepared between 1935 and 1939, "It cannot be assumed that the Red Cross in any future war would merely duplicate what it did in the World War."[1] Looking forward to the potential of future conflict and ARC action, labor shortages of the past had reportedly been replaced with a surplus of potential workers, and U.S. armed services had since developed more than adequate medical departments, thereby obviating the "necessity for much of the improvised, nonprofessional, volunteer and paid services which were necessary in the World War."[2] From ARC units of medical volunteers sent abroad, its defining activity and institutional identity had shifted.

However, the reputation of the Red Cross established in World War I provided both an inspiration to the founders of the AMBASD and ABMAC and an expectation of action that was not, ultimately, pursued. To the activists of the AMBASD, Red Cross attempts to remain neutral became a conservative statement, implicitly supporting Nationalist forces. For those behind the ABMAC, ARC inaction in the name of neutrality became an embodiment of insular American prejudice and racism. Either way, while offering a model for the aspirations of new units of private volunteers, the perceived lack of Red Cross action turned the institution's "neutrality" into affiliation with the enemy.

The Roots of the Red Cross

Although the abbreviated name of the "Red Cross" has become a household term in international aid, it is somewhat misleading in suggesting organizational unity. The Red Cross developed as a constellation of national societies affiliated by their symbolic representation and commitment to the Geneva Conventions. In fact, the loose coalition of Red Cross societies and the international committee itself offers a valuable historical parallel to the development of the private medical relief efforts that have become the subject of this study, and an integral part of their story.[3] Like the organizations of this study, the roots of the ICRC lay in a response to conflict. However, while growing out of the basic critique that military medical services were insufficient, the development of both the ICRC in Geneva and its affiliated national societies also remained closely tied to national identities, despite the ICRC's more international agenda. The ICRC saw cooperation with government and military structures as fundamental.[4] Hence while the ICRC sought to carve a legitimate space for itself through the creation of a new body of international humanitarian law, national Red Cross societies sought to bridge private action and governmental legitimacy as quasi-governmental entities.[5] By the end of World War I, most states formally recognized their national Red Cross societies as auxiliaries to national military medical forces.[6] While the "true test of philanthropy" for the 1860s Red Cross society may have lay in its assistance of the wounded enemy soldier, the highest ideal of the Red Cross society in World War I shifted toward its ability to mobilize national spirit in support of one's own troops and those of one's allies. Much like the organizations of this study, the Red Cross model did not promote pacifism or attempt to abolish war—its humanitarian interest lay, instead, in mitigating war's costs.

As throughout the Red Cross, World War I marked a turning point in ARC history. In 1918, the ARC counted one third of the U.S. population among its membership—including twenty million adult members and eleven million youth members. From a small, private organization largely dependent on the enthusiasm of its founder, Clara Barton, involvement in the ARC became both a patriotic duty and powerful tool of American diplomacy that offered an "alternative definition of American nationalism" in contrast to "both American insularity and militant liberal-capitalist interventions."[7] Receiving its first congressional charter in 1900, the ARC became the preferred relief organization of the U.S. government, with the responsibilities of fulfilling U.S. obligations to the Geneva Conventions, supporting the U.S. military, and sustaining infrastructure for both national and international relief in times of peace.[8] In 1913, ARC ties with the federal government were strengthened when President Woodrow Wilson was named honorary president of the ARC.[9]

As the ARC gained an unofficial monopoly among relief organizations, the U.S. government found an ally in the private sector to pursue missions of cultural diplomacy on its behalf. As part of U.S. expansion in the Progressive Era, the new American international agenda as embodied by the rapid growth of the ARC as "a moral obligation and a universal social justice issue" also promised to differentiate the U.S. from previous imperial powers.[10] However, alongside America's "Wilsonian moment" of internationalism, the momentum of the ARC's expansion peaked in 1918.[11] While involved in some post-war reconstruction and relief efforts, its activity abroad steadily diminished over the course of the interwar period.

Identity in Crisis: The Red Cross in the Interwar Years

Following the enormous expansion of Red Cross activity during World War I, the ICRC also faced challenges in the decades that followed. As Huber observed in 1934, "The impetuous growth of international ideas brought about a curious situation for the Red Cross," leading to the loss of "its former position as a kind of isolated headland in international life" and suddenly opening "the Red Cross movement itself and all its accomplished service . . . to question."[12] After the horrors of World War I, some questioned the implicit approval of war by the Red Cross as a function of international relations. Those with more pacifist leanings argued that by simply placing "a humanitarian bridle upon war," both the Red Cross model and the Geneva Convention were fundamentally "based upon a false principle."[13] Other critics saw the postwar period not as a time to reconsider Red Cross wartime activity, but rather as an opportunity to expand its peacetime role. One of these critiques came in the form of American Henry P. Davison and the League of Red Cross Societies (LRCS), which challenged ICRC jurisdiction in the 1920s. Bolstered by the recent expansive successes of the ARC, and with the support of President Woodrow Wilson, Davison sought to supplant the ICRC with a new federation of Red Cross societies coordinated by the ARC and emphasizing the peacetime promotion of international health.[14] While Davison's LRCS ultimately fell short of its more expansive goals, he did add a new dimension to discussions of the scope and purpose of the Red Cross as an international body and helped to facilitate the development of a new sphere of Red Cross activities beyond the battlefield.

Outside of ARC activity, the U.S. government continued to show interest in the potential of aid to influence trajectories of conflict and of peace—particularly in the years immediately following World War I. In 1921 the American Relief Administration, in coordination with American Federated Russian Famine Relief (a private organization), organized U.S. aid to provide famine relief to Russia.[15] Although famine relief was not war relief, many of the U.S. architects of Russian famine relief saw its role as critical to the prevention of conflict, counteracting more radical political groups and the perceived threat of Russian Communism.[16] Famine relief to Russia was implicitly sanctioned by the U.S. government and funded with congressional approval, despite a developing foreign policy that emphasized keeping the country out of foreign entanglements.[17] Meanwhile, victims of natural disasters in East Asia also became recipients of U.S. government aid, with state-sponsored funds supplying relief to victims of the Japanese earthquake in 1923. Even in its more limited role compared to prior decades, the ARC also maintained interest in Asian disaster relief, supplying famine and flood relief to China in the 1920s.[18]

As debates over Red Cross identity in both peace and war simmered during the 1920s and 1930s, the ICRC faced more basic financial difficulties. At the International Red Cross Conference in London in 1938, Huber argued that Red Cross activity rested predominantly on its national societies, with the devaluation of the Swiss franc and consistent decline in contributions to the ICRC since 1928. Huber and his colleagues also struggled against the increasingly common national prioritization of domestic concerns over international ones. Where international interests captured attention, the attention was often partisan. As noted in April 1937, "The great obstacle to the success of our appeals is the desire of the public to forward aid solely to the party of its preference."[19] Meanwhile, smaller aid groups developing out of more partisan support were finding success. The result was concerning to Huber and the ICRC, who noted that the differences were becoming so great that "the idea of the Red Cross itself is in danger," as such groups had begun to "report directly to the government and ignore the national Red Cross Society."[20] The ICRC also lamented that these same groups "never fail to use the sign of the Red Cross on the white ground."[21] The symbol of the red cross had always been central to the organization's identity and operations, and the ICRC was highly defensive of its use.

The ARC faced similar challenges over both its finances and aspirations for neutrality. Over the first two years of the Spanish Civil War, the ARC donated nearly $60,000 to the ICRC for distribution, in addition to spending approximately $40,000 in emergency relief and repatriation expenses for American citizens stranded in Spain at the outset of the conflict. The ARC also supported the work of the American Friends Service Committee, acquiring sixty thousand barrels of flour to be distributed in Spain through American Quaker volunteers.[22] Like the International Committee, ARC officials observed that the Red Cross policy of strict impartiality "had the tendency to slow down gift giving . . . as many people prefer to contribute only to the side with which they sympathize."[23] Meanwhile, the ARC itself seemed reluctant to become more deeply involved. Reporting to the ICRC shortly after the outbreak of the war (and an initial $10,000 donation from the ARC, which it claimed would be all it could do), "The whole sentiment of the country is for keeping out of Europe, and in official and private circles the feeling is that we should not expose ourselves in any way that might involve us."[24]

Among activists, rumors swirled about ARC activities in Spain—or lack thereof. Not only was the reported absence of Red Cross personnel in Spain at issue, but there were also accusations of a Red Cross bias toward the Nationalist side.[25] ARC vice president Ernest J. Swift seemed to contradict such reports. Describing his visit to Spain in December 1938, Swift repeatedly revealed sympathies for the Republican government.[26] Returning to the U.S. resolved to "redouble" his efforts to offer relief to Spain's civilian population, Swift's own sympathies seemed to have little effect on the overall policy of the ARC, which continued to play a peripheral role in Spanish relief. The Spanish Civil War saw the beginning of a critical discourse about the ARC that would intensify in the years following World War II. Although some claims were exaggerations, many perceived the ARC as failing to act in accordance with its own purpose.[27] As dentist Zachary Stadt disparagingly wrote in an account of Spain published in the *Harvard Dental Record*, "As for the American Red Cross in Spain . . . the least said the better."[28] The noted lack of immunity accorded to the symbol of the red cross not only exemplified the new brutality of modern warfare, but it also reflected an organizational break with warfare of the previous half a century. The AMBASD thus saw itself filling a role left empty by the perceived failure of both the ARC and its larger umbrella organizations, the ICRC and LRCS.

The AMBASD: Political Humanitarians?

Where the Red Cross struggled to maintain its work in Spain under a rigid cloak of impartiality, the AMBASD seemed to have an unexpected advantage. Even as the group emphasized its role in providing purely humanitarian relief, it had a political dimension that the Red Cross lacked. When asked by a Spanish reporter whether the AMBASD was part of a political movement, Barsky was quoted as replying, "No, it is entirely without the boundaries of politics and is based on the democratic and humanitarian feelings of the people of the United States."[29] Democracy and humanitarianism were not only compatible, but inherently linked, and somehow beyond the political realm in arising from a basic interest in humanity. As Dr. Friedman, a volunteer with the AMBASD, similarly concluded, "Who can deny that the future of medicine is inextricably linked with the destiny of democracy?"Dr. Friedman, however, was more explicit in his belief that attempts "to separate medicine and politics" were fundamentally flawed.[30]

However, this unity in purpose between political and humanitarian beliefs was only selectively publicized by the AMBASD. Historian Rey García has argued that the fact that U.S. medical volunteers were becoming part of the Republican military medical services once in Spain was not well known and something AMBASD publicists very consciously "preferred to omit."[31] Certainly, many of the AMBASD's promotional materials emphasized civilian populations as recipients of aid. As one pamphlet urged, "More and more the crying need for medical attention to the women and children of Spain, as well as the combatants, becomes apparent."[32] Combatants here are included as a secondary priority, when in practice they were more likely the first. However, in the same pamphlet, supporters are also urged to contribute in order to "help to lessen the pain of those soldiers who fight to preserve the democracy of Spain, who die so bravely, and whose lives can be saved, if we can send a hospital caravan to the front."[33] As the war progressed, international medical units, such as those staffed by the AMBASD, only became more closely integrated with Republican military medical services.

However, in communication with the American media, volunteers seemed by and large forthright about their own sympathies in Spain. As written by Stadt in his own published account, "We who are of the American hospital have no doubt in our mind as to the services we are rendering and the cause which we are serving."[34] Most published accounts of AMBASD personnel openly reference the group's association with Loyalist forces, or at least express sympathy with them. Inaccurate or misleading statements did sometimes appear, particularly, it seems, in articles announcing volunteers' departures. For instance, when Dr. Frances Vanzant's departure was announced in the *Houston Post*, the American unit she was a part of was reported as going to serve refugees and the hundreds of thousands of Spanish children left homeless by the war.[35] The article announcing her return in the *Houston Press*, however, makes no attempt to gloss over her service "in the medical department of the Loyalist army" where she was reported as helping to "build the morale of a shattered people."[36]

Red Cross Responses to Spain

At other levels of Red Cross infrastructure, the war in Spain presented a challenge to the ICRC as an ostensibly internal conflict. The ICRC's jurisdiction in civil war was still a matter of debate. Although the tenth International Red Cross Conference, held in Geneva in 1921, had established the resolution that "all victims of civil war or revolutionary disturbances have, without any exception, a right to assistance," where such aid might come from was still subject to question as of 1938.[37] Governments in the midst of civil war might see the provision of relief to the victims of a rebel party as aiding lawbreakers in an unwelcome interference in national sovereignty. The 1921 conference concluded that the national society of the relevant country had the primary duty of relief work. If the national Red Cross society could not meet demands, the ICRC would then help, but only if both the government and insurgents accepted such assistance.

Within a few weeks of the Nationalist rebellion, the ICRC had arranged for a delegate from Geneva to travel to Spain to assess the situation. The ICRC had tried contacting the Spanish Red Cross to inquire whether "it desired the assistance of its sister Societies," but had received no response. The ICRC's relative readiness to become involved has led some historians to suggest that the ICRC saw the war in Spain as an opportunity for expanding its influence to civil conflicts.[38] The chosen delegate, Dr. Marcel Junod, had just completed a similar mission to Ethiopia following the Italian invasion. After Junod met with both Republican and Nationalist leaders, the ICRC sent a larger delegation of representatives to "protect the emblem of the Red Cross" and to "facilitate the humanitarian work of the Red Cross."[39] This work, however, turned out to be of limited duration and scope as the ICRC struggled to maintain sufficient funds for its activities.

Its chronic lack of funds finally forced the ICRC to reexamine its policy of refusing unilateral gifts. Although wary of accepting "gifts with political significance," the ICRC decided that it would have to accept gifts destined for one side or the other—hoping that they would come in almost equal proportions, or at least proportions that could be equalized. This change in policy was not, however, widely publicized given the "truly delicate" status of the ICRC's operation in Spain.[40] And despite this concession, the ICRC continued to face serious financial limitations. By February of 1938, the ICRC had little choice but to scale back its activities. That month the ICRC announced that the six delegations working in Republican and Nationalist territory would be reduced to four, and then two—one for the government in Barcelona, the other for the nationalists in San Sebastian.[41] During the first years of the war, these delegations had been working with the two Spanish national societies (both the Nationalists and Republicans had their own Red Cross society) and the ICRC headquarters in Geneva to distribute donations of food and medical supplies, operate a family news service, help evacuate and repatriate refugees and internationals, provide prison relief, and facilitate prisoner exchanges.

As the war had progressed, pressure from the State Department and eventually Roosevelt himself had led the ARC to some action in collaboration through other groups—but these remained largely limited in scope. The Committee for Impartial Civilian Relief in Spain, headed by a prominent Catholic layman at Roosevelt's request, set the goal of raising $300,000 to finance the work of the ARC and Friends Service Committee in distributing flour. A storm of protest, however, reportedly followed. When Catholics claimed that such work was only a move to give aid to Loyalists, in connection with efforts to lift the embargo on munitions exports, the committee redirected one shipment, in February 1939, directly to the Nationalists. This, in turn, drew outrage from anti-Fascists following reports that Franco had been sending flour and wheat to Nazi Germany. The committee (again, a private committee with, it seems, connections to the U.S. government) was ultimately only able to raise $50,000 of its $300,000 goal before shutting down. By the end of the war, Nationalist leaders of the Spanish Red Cross reached out to the ARC for American assistance in repatriating Spanish refugees from France. Within the ARC, however, there was reluctance surrounding the real "neutrality" of the new Spanish Red Cross society and a hesitance to donate even just a few thousand dollars.[42]

The Red Cross and War in China

When war broke out in China, the ICRC found itself in a compromised position. If the ICRC had struggled to mount an effective response to problems in its own European backyard, China posed an even more remote reality. What limited ICRC action had been successfully pursued in Spain seemed to have been largely dependent on previously rare, spontaneous "private collections" and a special "bond between the Spanish populations of the Old and New worlds."[43] As in Spain, the ICRC first sent delegates to assess the developing situation. Along the northern Chinese front, ICRC representative Colonel C. E. De Watteville estimated that by November 1937 there had been at least eight hundred thousand casualties.[44] ICRC representatives continued sending reports into 1938, when Dr. Robert McClure (Canadian medical missionary, director of the Friends Ambulance Unit, and reporter to the ICRC) offered a promising assessment of China's potential.[45] Other ICRC representatives took a less optimistic view of both the war and the ICRC's role in it. When the British Evert Barger and Philip Wright traveled to northern China on the ICRC's behalf in 1941, they concluded that the committee "by reason of its narrow horizon and its unwillingness . . . to adapt itself to changing conditions, cannot be a channel through which Red Cross assistance from abroad can be effectively given."[46] Instead, Barger and Wright resigned from the ICRC to devote themselves to "a more effective form of foreign assistance."[47]

Outside of the ICRC, Huber noted that only two national societies took action of any significance in China. These two national societies had managed to collect—"partly, it must be owned, in association with other organizations—donations more than twice exceeding the sums contributed for help in Spain," in half the amount of time.[48] Although the founding vision of the Red Cross network had been largely Eurocentric, China was a signatory to the 1864 Geneva Convention and had established the first Chinese Red Cross Society (CRC) on 6 December 1899. As Caroline Reeves has argued, this development was a conscientious "diplomatic maneuver" by which China sought admittance to the internationally accepted "ranks of the civilized."[49] Now, the CRC had "all by itself . . . furnished 80% of the funds placed at the International Committee's disposal," funding the placement of an ICRC delegate in China for about six months.[50] While Huber failed to name the second recipient of his praise, the ARC seems a likely candidate. Reflecting on what lessons might be learned from the relative failures and successes of fundraising for Spain and China, he concluded that the "situation of foreign residents" with "powerful financial connections in Europe and the United States" had "played an essential part in the success of the collections" made for China.[51]

When fighting initially broke out between China and Japan in the summer of 1937, the ARC expressed little interest in extending itself into Asian affairs. In early September of that year, the ARC made the tentative announcement that it "might accept contributions for relief work in China" but that it did "not contemplate sending personnel to China or launching a national campaign."[52] In the wake of this announcement, several local chapters echoed such sentiments.[53] By the end of September 1937, the ARC had reported plans to spend $100,000 on medical supplies and hospital equipment to send to China. The ARC had already orchestrated the spending of $30,000 to assist American citizens stranded by the war, with $10,000 coming from American diplomatic officials and $20,000 coming from the Philippine Red Cross Society.[54] Initially, the ARC took the standard approach of offering aid to the national societies of both sides. When their offer was accepted by the Chinese, but refused by the Japanese, the ARC chose to focus their efforts accordingly with contributions received.[55] However, the Central Committee doubted the American people cared enough about China to support a national fundraising campaign.

What responses the ARC did receive in the late summer and fall of 1937 came mostly from groups with preexisting connections to China. ARC chapters along the Pacific coast were some of the most active, with residents of San Francisco's Chinatown raising enough money to purchase supplies to equip three five-hundred–bed hospitals by October 1937.[56] Some residents of Baltimore, Maryland, also took an early interest in ARC efforts to improve conditions for the Chinese—both through the local Chinese-American population and a segment of the medical community of Johns Hopkins University School of Medicine.[57] "Without formal solicitation by the local Red Cross Chapter," Dr. G. Canby Robinson and sixteen of his colleagues collected $135.50 in donations to China to be sent through the ARC.[58] Despite the initiative shown by these early efforts, they admittedly had a relatively limited financial impact.

On 25 January 1938, President Franklin D. Roosevelt called upon the ARC to launch a national appeal for China's relief.[59] By this time, the ARC had transferred $181,000 to the U.S. ambassador in China to distribute.[60] Funds raised in the nascent national campaign were, ARC president admiral Cary T. Grayson announced, to be distributed in China by the American Advisory Committee.[61] While not exactly front-page news, Roosevelt's appeal to the ARC received a small, but enthusiastic press response in the weeks that followed. Commentators in both the *New York Times* and the *Washington Post* lauded the appeal, labeled by one as "unprecedented in American history" for proposing "assistance to civilians of one nation involved in a foreign war" and yet "not the less acute because . . . the result of a man-made disaster rather than the work of nature in a malevolent mood."[62] With Americans' proud history of generosity toward those in need, most coverage implied that the president's appeal would be quickly met. From first lady Eleanor Roosevelt to religious leaders of Hartford, Connecticut, the new mission laid out for the ARC earned vocal supporters, while existing private relief agencies promised to step back from their appeals in support of a more unified national effort under the ARC.[63] As one observer already involved in other private efforts observed, the ARC announcement "was received with enthusiasm" as "everyone recognizes that the Red Cross with its great organization and prestige could handle this problem far more effectively than any new organization created for the purpose."[64] One congressman even proposed a bill to appropriate $5 million in federal funds to send to China in support of the civilian victims of war.[65]

Initial enthusiasm for the ARC's appeal, however, did not translate well into funds. By the beginning of May, only $170,000 in public donations had been collected.[66] The ARC national convention in May 1938 concluded with the resolution that local chapters must take greater action to revive the flagging campaign. After additional prodding from Roosevelt, ARC chairman Norman Davis attempted to encourage more vigorous local action by setting chapter fundraising quotas and announcing a new deadline of 15 June to meet the $1 million goal.[67] But even calls to donate on behalf of a world "challenged by the forces of paganism and barbarism" in which "huns and vandals" were "in the saddle again" and threatening the very foundation of civilization did not seem to be enough to turn the ARC's campaign around.[68] Finally, on 16 June 1938, the China Relief Drive was officially called off, having only collected $200,000 in public contributions since Roosevelt's initial appeal.[69]

Why did the ARC meet such resistance to this appeal for China? As Red Cross historian Foster Rhea Dulles later claimed, the China campaign was the first time an ARC campaign had met total failure.[70] Dulles argued that the ARC appeal had, from the start, been a half-hearted attempt, strongly resisted by the Central Committee, which anticipated trouble mobilizing an apathetic public from the very beginning. The replacement of ARC chairman admiral Cary Grayson following his death in 1938 with Norman Davis does not seem to have changed much at the national headquarters. ARC chapters reportedly followed the Central Committee's lead in taking a passive approach. Some claimed to have "received no instructions," while others reported having "no intention of conducting a campaign" beyond forwarding any contributions they received.[71] Such reports back up other contemporary observations over a basically disorganized campaign in which "the plea of the

Red Cross for funds was not generally understood" and had not been "put up to various organizations and churches and individuals as it should have been."[72]

Interestingly, the ARC's account of its activities in 1938 is recorded with marked differences. In a 1943 report summarizing ARC activities in China since 1937, there is no direct reference to any campaign failure. Instead, in the timeline of ARC activity, the following was reported:

> Following the President's appeal in January for $1,000,000 for China, the American National Red Cross made an additional appropriation of $100,000 and endeavored to stimulate public interest in the relief fund. Chapters were later placed on a quota basis. All red cross funds were transmitted to the Department of State and transferred through official channels to the American Advisory Committee composed of representative Americans resident in Shanghai. The committee allotted the funds to well established organizations including hospitals and refugee centers. As of June 30, 1938, the total amount of money made available was $629,454.02.[73]

In fact, the final figure cited by James Gwin in this report is substantially larger than the $200,000 reported in the *New York Times* on 16 June 1938.[74] The source of this discrepancy is unclear. The next chapter of Gwin's report jumps to nearly a year later, without further comment. Also excluded from the ARC's report was the rising involvement of other private relief organizations during this period. In May 1938, the ABMAC received a $25,000 anonymous donation, and in June 1938 (just as the ARC drive was being called off), China Civilian Relief collected $52,842. Such figures suggest a more complex cultural and political dynamic at play than more traditional explanations of an isolationist America.

The Chinese Red Cross Society

In China, the CRC faced its own challenges. Serving the medical needs of a country of China's population and size was no small feat. With China's army reportedly lacking a complete medical division at the start of the war, the CRC confronted the task of administering to a fighting force of about three million soldiers on active duty over a front of two thousand miles. Even still, both the military and the CRC faced severe shortages of manpower, with suggestions of there being no more than "barely 6,000 qualified and 3,000 'irregular' doctors nationwide."[75] Although the CRC had

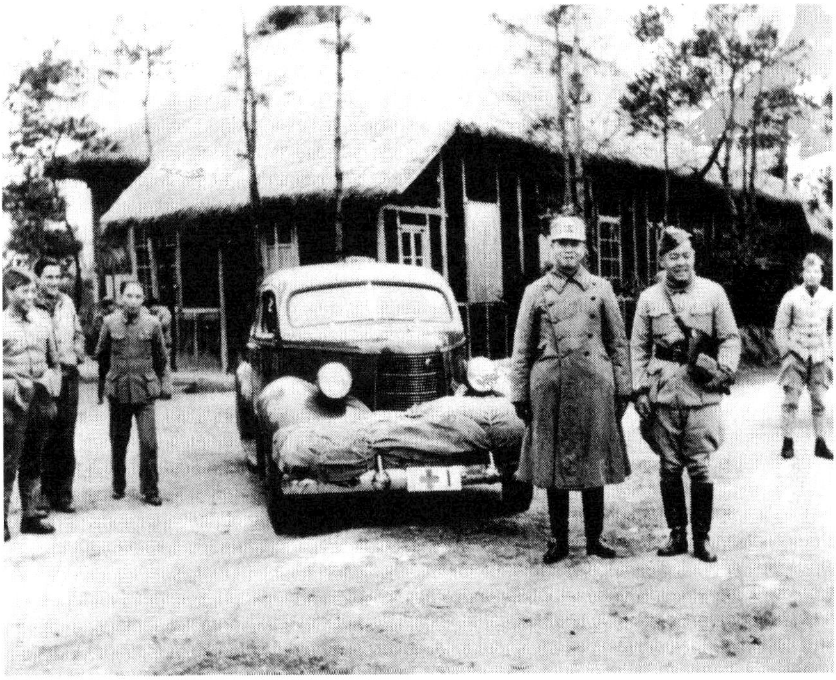

Figure 7. Dr. Robert Kho-Seng Lim (front right) smiling with members of the Chinese Red Cross Emergency Medical Training School in China (USC Records, Mudd Manuscript Library, Princeton University).

expanded significantly beyond its turn-of-the-century roots, opening hospitals in Shanghai and a number of other cities and incorporating the founding of over three hundred Red Cross chapters nationwide, the outbreak of war presented an even greater challenge.[76]

To respond to the challenge posed by China's new military enterprise, the CRC organized the Medical Relief Corps (MRC). Designed to address shortages of medical personnel in the Chinese army, by March of 1941 the MRC had established one hundred fifty medical units and grouped them according to nine "war areas."[77] Each group had instructions to cooperate with the nearest branch of the Army Medical Service, Emergency Medical Service Training School, and civil Public Health Department.[78] As described in a 1941 report, the MRC sought to "strengthen the Army Medical Service technically" as an "auxiliary to the Army Medical Service (as provided for by the Geneva Convention)" whose personnel worked "under the direction of the Army Medical Administration."[79]

Dr. Robert Kho-Seng Lim assumed leadership of the MRC in 1933. Born to Chinese parents in Singapore in 1897, Lim had a global upbringing. At the age of eight, Lim begin his education abroad in Scotland, coloring his English with a Scottish brogue for the rest of his life. When war broke out in Europe, he volunteered in France, where he was assigned to the Indian army as a warrant officer.[80] After the war, Lim returned to Scotland, completing his medical degree at Edinburgh University in 1919. Several years later, Lim won a fellowship through the China Medical Board to spend a year of research at the University of Chicago's Department of Physiology.[81] After returning to China, Lim joined the faculty of the PUMC. Lim's public career in China took off in the 1930s, during which time he became president of the Chinese Medical Association, chairman of the North China Council for Rural Reconstruction, and president of the CRC.[82]

Under Lim's leadership, the MRC and CRC underwent significant expansion. By 1940, the MRC had grown from twelve units attempting to cover twenty thousand Chinese soldiers to forty-nine units. In that same time, Lim also helped found a school designed to train two hundred men a month to become hospital attendants and stretcher-bearers. Lim later helped establish a hospital at Kweiyang, which became the largest medical center in wartime China. Medical education had become one of Lim's central concerns, and he pressed the PUMC to expand their educational programs in light of China's medical needs. The PUMC, however, remained firm in their mission of training leaders in medical education rather than lower level health care providers. With Lim's own career taking off in a different direction, he left the PUMC faculty and in 1941 was appointed inspector general of China's Medical Service.[83]

CRC Connections with the U.S.

Lim's initiative and talent in developing the Chinese Red Cross MRC was supplemented by his extensive international contacts. During the war, he helped the CRC build substantial support abroad through avenues outside of traditional Red Cross networks. One of Lim's well-established contacts in the U.S. was Harvard Medical School's Walter B. Cannon. In Cannon, Lim found both a loyal friend and a fervent supporter. Commenting to the popular American magazine *Reader's Digest* in 1939, Cannon depicted Lim as central to his own involvement in American relief to China. According to Cannon, "My own willingness to be a sponsor of ABMAC rests upon my thorough confidence in Dr. Lim's honesty and efficiency."[84]

A professor of physiology, Cannon became a prominent medical figure in the 1930s for his research in physiology and for his increasingly vocal role in international humanitarian work. His most famous contribution to physiology was in his development of the concept of homeostasis. Having volunteered with the ARC during World War I, however, Cannon also played a critical role in collaborative research with the British and Canadian armies on the problem of wound shock.[85] Cannon's work earned him invitations to visit fellow physicians and scientists all over the world. These professional friendships seemed to prove substantial inspiration for his work in international medical relief.

Encouraged by his personal relationship with fellow physiologist, Dr. Juan Negrín (leader of the Spanish Second Republic during the war), Spain became a particular concern of Cannon's in the 1930s. Following the establishment of the AMBASD, Cannon became a vocal supporter. However, Negrín and Cannon's relationship dated from much earlier. Following Negrín's studies at the Physiology Institute in Leipzig, Germany (terminated early because of World War I), Negrín planned to spend two years working in the U.S. with Cannon.[86] But Negrín's path led him back to Spain, where he became director of the newly established Laboratory of General Physiology, established by the same institute that had funded his studies abroad.[87]

Cannon's friendship with Lim dated from the early 1930s, when the two began sharing academic papers regarding their respective work in the field of physiology.[88] When Cannon's daughter, Wilma, moved to China with her then-fiancé John K. Fairbank in the early 1930s, Lim extended a warm welcome to the new couple.[89] Cannon himself later spent three months in China as a visiting professor at the PUMC, further solidifying his friendship with Lim.[90] Back in the U.S., Cannon's first foray into American relief to China came through the New England Committee for Relief in China. Chaired by Karl T. Compton, the New England Committee was one of the many grassroots relief efforts that had coalesced in the wake of the war in China. By the time President Roosevelt announced his challenge to the ARC to raise funds for China, the New England Committee had raised about $700.[91] Yielding to the anticipated ARC effort, the group called off their active appeal. However, within a few months Cannon wrote, "I learned, to my chagrin, that the Red Cross was making no important effort and was largely a receiving organization taking contributions which came to it."[92] Cannon wrote to President Roosevelt himself, questioning the passivity of the ARC's actions and reminding him of Chinese support to the U.S. during World

War I.[93] A similar letter from the New England Committee was even more direct, appealing to Roosevelt to use his "great influence . . . to induce the Red Cross to undertake this campaign actively."[94] Roosevelt wrote back to assure Cannon that "the meagre response to the appeal has been a matter of great concern to the officials of the Red Cross and they are endeavouring in various ways to secure a more active participation of the public," while also suggesting that "the Red Cross would see no necessity for your committee to discontinue its campaign."[95]

In the spring of 1939, Cannon became an official sponsor of the ABMAC, helping Marian Exter—who had also been involved in Spanish relief through the AMBASD—establish a Boston chapter for the organization.[96] Like the New England Committee, ABMAC leadership had similar expectations of ARC involvement. As described by Co Tui in 1939:

> The friends of China looked to the American Red Cross for action. This was natural since in sudden emergencies the machinery of the American Red Cross were the most effective and in the second place to form an organization for Chinese relief would mean months of delay . . . There was a delay of months before the American Red Cross acted. The progressives were preoccupied with Spain and other European crises. The result was that while the Chinese communities poured forth their money, the response from the American public was very meagre.[97]

Co Tui placed the origins of the ABMAC in both the existence of an active and concerned community of Chinese-Americans and "friends of China," and a perceived failure of Red Cross action. The ABMAC's perception of supplanting a lacking ARC effort is echoed in the ABMAC's own relationship with the CRC. Lim and Co Tui corresponded extensively early in the war, and Co Tui helped raise money for the CRC through his own organization. In 1940, the relationship between the two was recognized in a certificate from the National Red Cross Society of China unequivocally naming the ABMAC "their fully accredited representatives in the United States of America, for the purpose of securing medical supplies, raising funds, and making better known the activities of the National Red Cross Society of China, among friends, sympathizers, and humanitarians in that great country."[98] Even after the ARC began taking a more active role, the ABMAC remained an official representative of the CRC.[99]

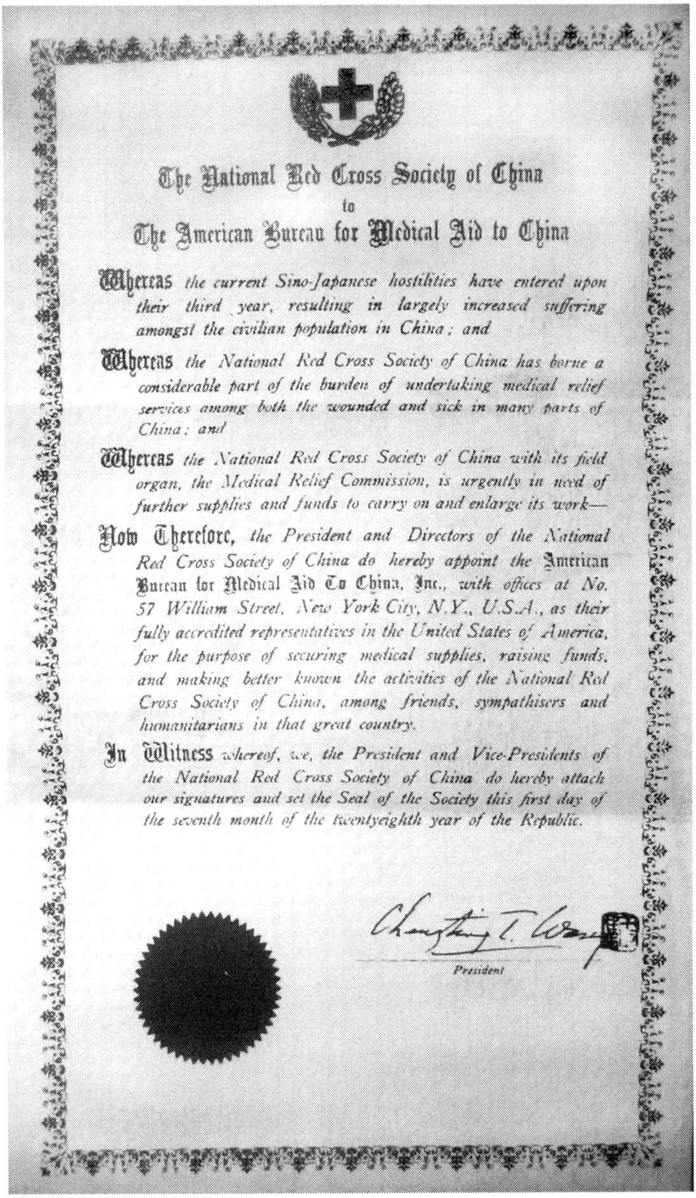

The National Red Cross Society of China
to
The American Bureau for Medical Aid to China

Whereas *the current Sino-Japanese hostilities have entered upon their third year, resulting in largely increased suffering amongst the civilian population in China; and*

Whereas *the National Red Cross Society of China has borne a considerable part of the burden of undertaking medical relief services among both the wounded and sick in many parts of China; and*

Whereas *the National Red Cross Society of China with its field organ, the Medical Relief Commission, is urgently in need of further supplies and funds to carry on and enlarge its work—*

Now Therefore, *the President and Directors of the National Red Cross Society of China do hereby appoint the* American Bureau for Medical Aid To China, Inc., *with offices at No. 57 William Street, New York City, N.Y., U.S.A., as their fully accredited representatives in the United States of America, for the purpose of securing medical supplies, raising funds, and making better known the activities of the National Red Cross Society of China, among friends, sympathisers and humanitarians in that great country.*

In Witness *whereof, we, the President and Vice-Presidents of the National Red Cross Society of China do hereby attach our signatures and set the Seal of the Society this first day of the seventh month of the twentyeighth year of the Republic.*

President

Figure 8. Certificate from the National Red Cross Society of China to the American Bureau for Medical Aid to China, 1940 (ABMAC Records, Rare Book and Manuscript Library, Columbia University).

Lim's role in CRC leadership, however, also led to friction. In February 1943, Lim was the target of a Chinese government investigation for misuse of funds.[100] Although ultimately cleared of all charges, the controversy led to a major reorganization of CRC leadership. The result left Lim in a more peripheral position as technical advisor, with Dr. Chiang Monlin in the role of the presidency.[101] From the perspective of one American observer, the conflict arose "largely based on personal animosities and mutual distrust."[102] Not all shared the ABMAC's high opinion of Lim. In the midst of the controversy, UCR field representative Dwight W. Edwards revealed doubts over Lim's capability as a leader, despite his other professional talents.[103] When debates over supporting Lim and the EMSTS arose, these conflicting viewpoints led to substantial disagreements between the ABMAC and UCR.

Although the ABMAC sought to portray itself as the primary American representative of the CRC, it was not the only private organization in the U.S. acting in support of the CRC. In August 1938, CAC director Oliver Haskell reported to Dr. Robert Lim, then leader of the CRC, that a citizens committee in Buffalo had raised $1,000 for the CRC—and that the CAC had plans of expanding such citizen committees.[104] Haskell and Lim continued to correspond through the fall of 1938 regarding further donations to the CRC, in addition to coordinating the logistics of a handful of medical volunteers partially sponsored by the CAC. Early on, Haskell offered Lim his own analysis of the portrait of China relief in the U.S., particularly in reference to the controversy of the ARC:

> This [the ARC] is a very conservative, not to say reactionary, organization. They raised very little money for China because they didn't half try. They feel that they must be impartial in this war and not help China any more than they help Japan, even though Japan declined their aid. Thus it is impossible for us to get trucks or anything else from the Red Cross . . . It is important that you should understand that the American League for Peace and Democracy is influential mainly among left wing groups. Thus, if it is desired to reach the Red Cross or the United Council for Civilian Relief in China it should be done through Chinese diplomatic channels, either official or unofficial. We can bring pressure to bear on them only very indirectly.[105]

Nevertheless, the CAC continued to supply the CRC with funds, earmarked for the Northwest. Reporting to Haskell at the end of September,

Lim acknowledged the receipt of another $1,500 donation, noting "We have sent the whole amount to the 8th route army headquarters . . . through Miss Agnes Smedley for the use of the Reserve Field Hospital."[106] CAC donations to the CRC were also channeled to Dr. Bethune in support of his work. By September 1938, Dr. Lim reported that over $70,000 in supplies had been sent to medical services in northwest China.[107]

While predominantly staffed by Chinese, a handful of Western volunteers did appear among the Red Cross Units of the Northwest. Arranging the arrival of several medical volunteers was one of the CAC's first activities, arranged by Haskell and Lim in the late summer and fall of 1938. By 5 September 1938, Jean Ewen had arrived in Yenan and was on her way to southern Shansi, where she was to join the Red Cross units (and two other Canadian volunteers, Dr. Norman Bethune and Dr. Richard Brown) attached to General Chu Teh's army.[108] Located about four hundred kilometers north of Xian (Shensi), Yenan had become the headquarters of the former Red Army and regional government seat—in addition to a base for several CRC units and the League of Nations Epidemic Commission.[109] When the local population swelled from three thousand to 30,000, caves replaced houses as shelter for the influx of refugees. The "border hospital" (formerly the Red Army Central Hospital) in Yenan followed the same model, and the "cave hospital" of the Northwest became a popular public interest story for CAC fundraising appeals at home.

In early October 1938, direct communication between Haskell and Lim seems to have shifted, with the China Defence League becoming the main intermediary between the CAC and China. From that month onwards, all funds directed to the CRC Society from the CAC were to be transmitted by the China Defence League.[110] Meanwhile, the ABMAC's connection with Lim and the CRC Society continued to grow stronger.[111] The ARC, too, continued to have a presence in China. Despite the failure of its 1938 campaign, correspondence dating from 1938 and 1939 suggests it was involved in arranging the shipment of several sizeable donations of pharmaceuticals to China.[112] Such shipments do not appear to have been publicized, however, and the ARC continued to receive letters of complaint in 1939 and 1940 from private citizens who felt that the ARC was not living up to its responsibility as a representative of the U.S. in the global arena.[113]

A closer examination of ARC records negates both Dulles's claim that the ARC's interest in China was not resurrected until after U.S. entry into World War II and many of the charges laid against it by private citizens. Of course, with the ARC still closely tied to the U.S. government as a quasi-state apparatus, its activities multiplied after the U.S. entered the war, with the concentration of its activities in China peaking between 1943 and 1946. However, by 1940 ARC activities in China rivaled those of smaller private groups. That year, for example, the ARC purchased and shipped five million tablets of quinine to the CRC, while the ABMAC continued fundraising for a third shipment of one million tablets of quinine. Although perhaps lacking some of the enthusiasm of ABMAC leadership, the ARC still seemed to maintain some advantage in the scale of potential funding available for its work.[114]

In the autumn of 1940, the ARC sent its first delegation of ARC representatives to oversee the group's work in China. Dr. John Earle Baker and Mr. Walter Wesselius contributed to the establishment of three bases for ARC operation in Shanghai, Hong Kong, and Kunming (later to be moved to Chungking).[115] Within six months of the arrival of Baker and Wesselius in China, the CRC appealed to the ARC for funds to support its Medical Relief Corps. By the end of the summer of 1941, the ARC agreed to fund the $707,000 for one year of the organization's supply and transport needs.[116] But that amount was only a fraction of the ARC's financial commitment to China that year. In 1941, ARC reports record shipping $3,909,937.82 in supplies purchased both by government and ARC funds.[117] By 1942 the ARC's activities had expanded to the extent that a directory of personnel in China was created. This directory consisted primarily of Americans already present in China, whether as diplomatic staff, members of U.S. missions, military personnel, or private businessmen, in addition to prominent Chinese working in state, military, or welfare institutions.[118]

While the ARC's renewed commitment to the CRC challenged the ABMAC's claim to representing CRC interests in the U.S., it did not displace the organization entirely. As ARC activities expanded, ARC and ABMAC officials agreed to a plan that would leave both organizations active without a duplication of effort. While the ABMAC had carried out most of its activities between 1937 and 1940 through the CRC Medical Relief Corps, from 1941 onward, the ABMAC directed increasing amounts of its attention elsewhere.[119] In particular, this period marked a shift toward medical education through the support of Lim's Emergency Medical Service Training Schools and the establishment of an Army Nursing School.[120] Although the ABMAC retained a titular claim to being the CRC's "official representative" in the

U.S., the ARC requested that the ABMAC not use the name of the CRC in its fundraising work.[121] Any hesitance in getting involved in China aid appears to have begun to fade as the ARC attempted to reestablish primacy in dealings with its sister society in China.

Mobilization for World War II contributed to the expansion of ARC activities in 1940, almost without reference to the 1938 campaign. A later ARC report cited a continuous chain of work in China, without reference to the 1938 campaign. Instead, reports of the logistical challenges of moving supplies into China dominated ARC accounts. The Burma Road had, for a time, seemed to provide and imperfect solution, cutting 717 miles through roughly mountainous landscapes in a winding, one-way road.[122] The closure for three months in 1940 by Great Britain in response to Japanese diplomatic pressure foreshadowed the more permanent closure to allied forces following the Japanese occupation of Burma in 1942. Following this more permanent closure, the only way for supplies based in India to make their way into the war zone in China was by air, and the U.S. Army made space for numerous shipments of ARC supplies to enter China on their flights. Nevertheless, the limited space available often prioritized medical supplies for combatants over civilian needs.[123] As the global dimensions of the war expanded, the debate between civilian and combatant needs intensified. Furthermore, the presence of U.S. military forces in China, with access to a vastly different scale of transportation resources, left the ARC in a prime position to organize the distribution of aid as a paramilitary organization, even after other institutions such as the UNRRA entered the picture.[124]

Even before formally entering the war, the U.S. government had begun to move away from more isolationist policies through aid short of war. On 11 March 1941, President Roosevelt signed the Lend-Lease Act, formally ending the pretense of American neutrality. Although initially constructed to offer material assistance to Great Britain, in April the policy was extended to China. Among other things, this extension supplied Lim with much-needed fuel for the Chinese Red Cross MRC.[125] That same year saw the passage of the Emergency Relief Appropriation Act, which promised $50 million for the "relief of refugee men, women, and children who have been driven from their homes or otherwise rendered destitute by hostilities or invasion," for "agricultural, medical, and other relief supplies to be distributed through the American Red Cross or such other agencies as the President might designate."[126] On 17 December 1941, ten days after the Japanese attack on Pearl

Harbor, the Third Supplemental National Defense Appropriation Act authorized an additional $35 million for relief efforts.[127] As the U.S. mobilized for war, new governmental structures multiplied in an effort to accommodate, encourage, and, ultimately, wield some control over the equally proliferating local and transnational networks of aid.

Conclusions

By the 1930s, institutions such as the ICRC and its affiliated national societies had become well-established leaders in the realm of medical relief in times of war.[128] In the U.S., the ARC had expanded beyond national boundaries, developing a unique tradition of activity in China over the first three decades of the twentieth century.[129] A closer examination of Red Cross responses reveals a parallel perspective from which to examine the development of private American relief efforts to Spain and China in the late 1930s. As examples of a developing tradition of private medical activism in the interwar period, such grassroots efforts engaged in a complex interaction with evolving Red Cross responses. When initial ICRC and ARC responses fell short of expectations in responding to the Spanish Civil War and Second Sino-Japanese War, organizations such as the AMBASD, ABMAC, and CAC gained strength. Seemingly based on their stricter claims of neutrality, the ARC struggled in what fundraising efforts it did make during this period—and the ARC's campaign for China was initially called off following inadequate donations. However, the trajectories of the new private aid groups depended heavily on responses of the U.S. government, whose foreign policy interests did not always match with the political interests of these humanitarian activists. U.S. policy toward Spain, for instance, would never meet the expectations of the more politically motivated constituents of the AMBASD. Meanwhile, those supporting American assistance to the Chinese would soon find their interests aligning with those of the U.S. government.

CHAPTER THREE

Defining Aid
Private Interests Meet the State

When the AMBASD began to send personnel abroad to Spain, the U.S. State Department wavered on its response to these private efforts in light of U.S. neutrality legislation. By the time the ABMAC and CAC began organizing aid to China under UCR, the U.S. government had reestablished a more proactive stance in regulating and supporting aid abroad. Their actions supporting China and its military offered a positive tool to U.S. interests on multiple levels, and groups under UCR found a powerful ally in the state. These alliances cannot be summarized simply as a product of citizen activism successfully lobbying a change in government policy, or as an example of the U.S. government actively seeking allies in a policy course it had already set. While the U.S. government remained, in many ways, the more powerful institution in the equation (at the very least in terms of financial resources), navigating the interactions between these groups was a process of give-and-take between private groups and state resources.

Since the post-World War I wave of humanitarian activity seeking to help war-torn areas recover and prevent future conflict, the early 1930s saw a step back from such expansive international efforts conducted by the state. With the rise of private activism and humanitarian action at the end of the 1930s, however, the U.S. government renewed its interest in reconfiguring such efforts to support new developments in U.S. foreign policy. These interests began to be re-awakened in U.S. State Department debates over its policy toward AMBASD medical volunteers in light of the prohibition it had placed on U.S. citizens traveling to Spain in general. Such travel restrictions had been enforced under U.S. neutrality legislation, although debates over statutes prohibiting the enlistment of U.S. citizens in foreign armies were also cited. However, AMBASD volunteers managed to tread a fine line in their activities, which in practice often contradicted U.S. foreign policy at the time. While travel restrictions for China were also initially enforced, by the time UCR was established, it had found a significant ally in U.S. government institutions of aid.

The Controversy of the AMBASD

In first contacting the Department of State's Passport Division, the AMBASD presented their work directly. Following a meeting with Dr. Miller in early December 1936, a Passport Division representative reported, "I asked him if they would take care of non-combatants in other areas and he said, no, that the sympathy of the his organization was for the Loyalist cause and they were attempting to aid the Loyalist cause by this move."[1] Writing to Secretary of State Cordell Hull on 31 December 1936, AMBASD chairman Walter B. Cannon stated, "The object of the Medical Division is to provide ambulance units, including medical supplies and personnel, to relieve the urgent need of wounded men in the armies of the Spanish Government."[2] While Cannon admitted that "the effort to mitigate suffering in the Loyalist armies is, in a sense . . . taking sides," he argued that the humanitarian dimension of their work was ultimately more significant.[3] For Cannon, the humanitarian qualities of the AMBASD's work incorporated the support (through the professional sphere of medicine) of the democratically elected Republican government.

Although the State Department, in response, appeared reluctant to either grant formal approval of the AMBASD's project or expressly forbid it, the first unit of AMBASD volunteers left for Spain unchallenged. While expressing sympathy with the "devastation" in Spain and "any proposals which may be made out to mitigate the terrible suffering of the Spanish people," the State Department emphasized the national policy of "the strictest non-interference in Spanish affairs" and the ARC's choice to avoid direct participation for these same reasons.[4] The State Department framed its objection to Cannon's inquiry by identifying the ARC as the only neutral (and congressionally approved) conduit for channeling aid and, as such, also the authority on humanitarian aid. This reaction became a stock response in the following months, as inquiries trickled in regarding the legality of the AMBASD's relief work in light of U.S. neutrality. A particularly interesting series of correspondence developed between the Chrysler Corporation and the State Department, discussing whether ambulances and personal armored cars would be considered military equipment or part of legal humanitarian aid.[5] At the heart of all these debates—and especially that of the humanitarian classification of the AMBASD—lay legal concerns surrounding statutes prohibiting U.S. citizens from serving in foreign armies. At least one Passport Division official argued that such concerns should be more of a concern for the Federal Bureau of Investigation (FBI) than a question for Passport Officials to decide.[6] Although this same assessment quoted the Geneva Convention of 1929 in stating that "a recognized society of a neutral country may only lend the services of its sanitary personnel and formations to a belligerent with the prior consent of its own Government and the authority of such belligerent"—yet still openly questioned whether Loyalist Spain would fall into that category.[7]

With news spreading of the first unit's arrival in Spain, requests for clarification of U.S. policy also began to arrive from the American Consulate in Barcelona. Citing a recent press release in January 1937, American consul general Mahlon F. Perkins wrote, "If the American citizens concerned are, as stated, actually proceeding 'for service with the Spanish Government,' I cannot see that the humanitarian nature of the service would render them immune from any penalties to which they might be liable under the provisions of the statutes mentioned."[8] Perkins continued, "Should it be felt, however, that such Americans are entitled to any more considerate treatment by this office than Americans bearing arms in service of the Spanish Government, I should very much appreciate receiving an expression of the Department's attitude toward a matter which may possibly become a somewhat perplexing practical question."[9] The State Department remained undecided on what their public stance would be.

Over the weeks that followed, Perkins continued sending updates on Spanish news coverage of the activities of AMBASD volunteers. On 12 February 1937, Perkins forwarded an article entitled "Empresa Humanitaria: La Misión Sanitaria de los Estados Unidos, en Barcelona," in which the author describes volunteer medical units from the U.S. as ultimately forming "part of the anti-fascist army."[10] As February wore on, the State Department continued to struggle with defining its policy. Finally, the State Department replied to Perkins with the telegrammed instructions (and rather unclear distinction) that "if members ambulance unit referred to form part of military forces they should be treated in same manner as members armed forces," but that "if merely attached to military forces in performance service humanitarian nature distinction may be drawn between them and members armed forces."[11]

Meanwhile, as the AMBASD prepared a second unit of volunteers for departure, the group ran into difficulties obtaining passports. On 13 February, the AMBASD telegrammed the State Department to report that passport officials had refused to grant passports to the group's four surgeons and six nurses, closing with the hope that they would "inform passport officials of correct policy."[12] Defending their actions to the State Department, a Passport

Division official suggested that the purpose of the AMBASD's work in Spain was "open to question." While admitting that an exception could be made for the group, the official argued that a refusal to issue passports to those intending to go to Spain would be more consistent with state policy. "However," the official warned, "if passports are refused there is in my opinion little doubt that this organization will do everything it can to bring unfavorable publicity upon the Department, basing it upon the refusal of the Department to maintain its tradition of extending humanitarian aid."[13] Within a couple of weeks, the State Department announced that no Americans would be granted permission to travel to Spain and, as of 3 March 1937, all Americans applying for passports would have to sign an affidavit confirming that they would not travel to Spain.[14] As predicted, however, this new policy triggered a string of letters of protest to the State Department, encouraged by the AMBASD.

The protests came from both individuals and organizations. Many came from physicians, who cited their professional standing in urging the government to reconsider its policy. The American Civil Liberties Union told the AMBASD that they were prepared to take a test case to court to overturn the department's decision, as they believed the ruling violated citizens' rights.[15] No legal battle proved necessary, however, as the State Department modified its stance by the end of March, conceding that passports to Spain would be issued to "physicians, nurses, and necessary attendants of bona fide medical and relief missions."[16] On 19 March 1937, Secretary of State Hull wrote directly to the American consulate at Havre, France, with a list of AMBASD volunteers who were to be permitted to enter Spain on U.S. passports.[17] This statement modified its earlier position, granting the only permissions to travel to Spain to "bona fide representatives of American newspapers duly assigned to Spain."[18] Under the new regulations, the AMBASD continued orchestrating the departure of a series of new volunteer units.

However, the question of whether or not AMBASD volunteers constituted a "bona fide medical and relief mission" continued to be debated within the State Department. This debate was fuelled both by continued reports from Perkins in Barcelona and an ongoing legal debate within the State Department in Washington, DC. On 20 April, Perkins forwarded two articles to the State Department announcing the arrival in Barcelona of a second and third unit of American medical volunteers. He gave his own assessment of the situation bluntly. "A survey of the facts," he wrote, "can leave no reasonable doubt that these expeditions have been sent to Spain not from purely humanitarian motives, but with the primary purpose of assisting one of the opposing parties to win the war."[19] Perkins suggested that the AMBASD could even be "lending more effective aid to the 'Government' than would an equal number of American citizens bearing arms." Although he admitted that such relatively small groups of volunteers would be unlikely to have a major impact in the final outcome of the war, Perkins saw problems with their presence in terms of U.S. neutrality. By advertising that "organized groups of Americans are leaving the United States to help what their opponents call the 'Red' or 'Communist' cause," he observed "their arrival . . . to create the belief that there is a bit of a sham about the 'complete neutrality of America.'"[20] Such questions saw further complications when at least six hundred passports of U.S. citizens volunteering in the International Brigades were reported as missing. By 1940, these missing passports had begun to be reported as appearing in the U.S.S.R. and Mexico for use by Communist Party members seeking to undermine the U.S. government.[21] Some Passport Division officials seemed to conclude that it was not the role of the Passport Division to police where applicants for passports were intending to go—and that such matters should be dealt with by other branches with respect to the statute prohibiting the enlistment of U.S. citizens in foreign armies.

Emerging from this debate are the problems and challenges that arose in the practical application of the term "humanitarian." While prioritizing combatants as the recipients of aid efforts echoed ARC efforts in World War I, such aid turned into a divisive contradiction of terms in the Spanish Civil War. AMBASD volunteers occupied an awkward space. While affiliation with Republican military forces directly contradicted ideals of a "neutral" endeavor, the practical dimensions of their work remained congruent with other accepted traditions of humanitarian aid in war.

The AMBASD as Humanitarian Organization

The composition of the AMBASD's executive committee and list of professional sponsors played a central role in the portrayal of their work at home. Cannon's leadership and the constituency of the national medical committee reinforced the image of the organization as one pursuing humanitarian—rather than political—work. As argued by historian Rey García, this differentiation was central to the organization's success.[22] The support of physicians was valuable in that they could be portrayed as acting solely in a professional capacity, looking to relieve human suffering without political designs. The medical volunteers in Spain similarly became "politically irreproachable" by their professions.[23]

A number of medical personnel became important advocates for the organization by offering accounts of their experiences in Spain. Publications ranging from local newspapers to political periodicals such as the *Daily Worker* printed letters from personnel in Spain, or interviews with volunteers who had recently returned home. Although the details and tone of these articles varied depending on the individual and news source, many shared common themes. Highlighted as first-hand accounts of the Spanish conflict, volunteers assumed roles of witnesses backed up by their professional status. Headlines such as "Doctor Serving at Spanish Frontier Tells of War Horror, Human Suffering" and "Red Cross Vanishing, Hospitals Now Targets, Says American Doctor" were common.[24] Such articles were valued as testimonials to the realities of war—realities made worse by the new and modern nature of warfare.

In the Spanish Civil War, as in other "modern" wars, the boundaries between military and civilian spheres became increasingly blurred.[25] Building from Max Weber's definition, modern warfare became defined by its technological innovation and bureaucratic organization.[26] The deviations from the previous rules of engagement also became a defining feature of the modern war—with particular relevance for the medical units treating the wounds that resulted. Reports of Fascist bombing of hospitals and ambulances appeared in a number of accounts. As quoted in one New York newspaper, Barsky reported, "The old days of using a red cross sign for protection in war are gone" as "the Fascists go for them with airplane bombs."[27] The use of exploding bullets was also cited as a deviation from the "established rules of warfare."[28] Such ammunition had been prohibited under the Hague Convention of 1899, but both Barsky and Fried reported observing their effects in human flesh in Spain. As Neugass later described, "A good clean bullet hole which enters one side of a man and comes out of the other is a rare luxury common only in the tranquility of the World War."[29] By Neugass's account, actions taken against medical units themselves were even worse than the technological aberrations of advancements in weaponry.[30]

Back at the American consulate in Spain, Perkins concluded his recommendations to the U.S. State Department by unequivocally stating that any concession to the department's passport policy on AMBASD volunteers on the grounds of humanitarian work was groundless. No matter how respectable the AMBASD's leadership at home may have been—and he admitted the organization's list of distinguished supporters was impressive and must sincerely believe in their cause—they were misinformed as to the reality of the situation in Spain, which oscillated between "tyranny" and "chaos." In many ways, Perkins's assessment provides a noteworthy reflection of U.S. attitudes toward the Spanish Civil War and the foundation for its foreign policy responding to the war. State policy, however, did not agree with all its constituents, and the AMBASD's action became as much a statement of dissent toward the U.S. government as an expression of solidarity with Republican Spain.

The AMBASD as a Political Group

In the aftermath of the outbreak of war, organizations dedicated to aiding Spain multiplied, with their political orientations echoing the coalition of liberal parties within the Popular Front. Beginning in May 1937, by congressional ruling, all organizations involved in relief work abroad had to register with the U.S. State Department. Twenty-six organizations registered for work in Spain, although three were responsible for nearly half of all relief sent from the U.S. to Spain.[31] Of these three, the North American Committee to Aid Spanish Democracy maintained strong ties with the United Front, while the Medical Bureau remained most closely connected with the U.S. Communist Party, and the Spanish-American United Spanish Societies to Aid Spain (USSAS) kept Socialist affiliations. The more broadly liberal American Friends of Spanish Democracy, which helped in the initial development of the Medical Bureau and North American Committee (which would later merge), became less influential as the conflict progressed. Such political differentiations were important factors in the relationships between these organizations at home. For instance, Communists and the North American Committee had, early on, refused to support the USSAS for reasons of both political affiliation and reports of excessively high overhead costs.[32]

Communist involvement in the AMBASD became a particularly strong point of controversy, both for contemporaries and historians since. From the perspective of organizational efficiency and success in achieving the group's humanitarian objectives, Communist Party involvement proved a mixed blessing. Political rivalries created an unstable public image that became a disincentive for more widespread support, in addition to leading to a potential waste of organizational energy and resources. However, as Smith points out, Communist infrastructure also facilitated the building of a nationwide network, as well as improving financial efficiency. As Smith's analysis of State Department records concludes, organizations with greater Communist links maintained lower administrative overheads and greater fiscal responsibility than non-Communist organizations. However, the problems posed by Communist links to public image in the U.S. outweighed the financial realities, and when the North American Committee and Medical Bureau merged in 1938 to become the most politically powerful organization of the Spanish aid groups, they also became a more visible target for criticism.

Smith also assesses the possible foundations of criticisms that such aid groups became siphons for funds to go directly to Communist Party interests and propaganda. One of his findings suggest that financial reports illustrating questionable overhead organizations did not account for non-cash donations.[33] Smith goes on to argue that a more thorough examination of organizational integrity and the real destinations of funds and supplies would require a more detailed examination of the International Coordinating Committee in Paris, which acted as liaison between international aid organizations and the Spanish government. Although largely beyond the scope of Smith's study (and as yet unexamined by other published research), Smith notes that a close examination of organization records in the U.S. confirms that the vast majority of donations appear to have made their way to Paris. Both Peter Rhodes, NAC liaison in Paris, and Sandor Voros (writing in a later period in which he had turned against the Communist Party) reinforce the organization's accountability in forwarding the donations received there to medical purposes in Spain.

Ultimately, while the AMBASD appears to have first begun as an independent organization, which maintained itself as separate from International Brigades in the recruitment of volunteers, the distinctions between the two groups grew murkier in Spain. Medical and military threads became further interwined when former volunteers of the AMBASD joined the veterans association of American International Brigade volunteers after the war. And some modern accounts do not differentiate the volunteers of the AMBASD from the International Brigades at all. For instance, the Spanish translation of Neugass's memoir is titled *La Guerra es Bella* (a direct translation of *War Is Beautiful*), with the subheading "*un brigadista internacional en la Guerra Civil Española*"—"an international brigader in the Spanish Civil War." Of course, many of the accounts describing the independent origins of the AMBASD were written in the height of the Cold War era, at a time when the FBI was investigating a number of volunteers. It may be impossible to say what effect, if any, this may have had on the retelling of the story by those who maintained a more independent nature of AMBASD.

United China Relief

With Spanish relief agencies in the U.S. (including the AMBASD) uniting under the North American Committee, the paths of the ABMAC and CAC merged with other China aid agencies under United China Relief (UCR). Officially incorporated in the state of New York in the early months of 1941, UCR became an umbrella organization for eight other relief groups working in medical, educational, and economic fields. However, despite facing similar challenges as the North American Committee in attempting to unite disparate interests in one organization, private American aid to China embarked on a very different trajectory to that of its Spanish cousin. Although many factors contributed to this difference, UCR's list of supporters probably helped.

Although the idea behind UCR did not belong to publishing magnate Henry R. Luce, his involvement—financially, logistically, and ideologically—played a critical role in the organization's early development. Luce contributed nearly $60,000 of his personal fortune to the organization between 1939 and 1941, and secured substantial individual contributions from a handful of other wealthy Americans, including Doris Duke (heiress to a family tobacco fortune) and Bernard Baruch (financier who headed the War Industries Board in World War I). Baruch made the largest single contribution in the organization's history, of $102,340 in 1942.[34] Nevertheless, most of UCR's funding in its first years came from small contributions. Considering UCR's objective of raising awareness and sympathy among the American public, this was seen as a highly positive development. As historian T. Christopher Jespersen has argued, the number of contributions became as important as the amount raised.

While Luce provided influential financial support, much of the impetus behind UCR seems to have come from Bettis A. Garside. Garside had a long-standing relationship with the Luce family through the American missionary community, and actually became the biographer of Henry Luce's father. Garside had lived in China for four years, joining the Presbyterian mission there in 1922 and also teaching education at Cheeloo University in Jinan. In response to the changing political situation in the Far East in the 1930s, Garside organized the American Committee for Non-Participation in Japanese Aggression in 1938, which advocated boycotts of Japanese goods and the prevention of shipments of scrap iron to Japan.[35] Collaborating with individuals such as Walter Judd, this group became the core of the later "China Lobby."[36]

UCR's Board of Directors became the command center for its operations.[37] Its initial objectives were planned in four parts. Firstly, UCR was to coordinate existing fundraising efforts. Secondly, it sought to become the primary distributor for the money raised in these efforts. Thirdly, it aimed to raise awareness among the American people about conditions in China. Finally, it sought to "reassure the Chinese people that the traditional American feelings of friendship and goodwill toward them persisted."[38] Within UCR, medical aid became only one piece of a larger expression of American goodwill. Through its eight member agencies, it was active in five fields: medicine and health, child welfare, education, disaster relief, and economic reconstruction. To accomplish the objectives, the board of directors set a three-stage plan to raise $5 million in its first year, as it simultaneously transitioned leadership from member agencies to the central organization.

Drawing from the resources of Luce's media empire, which often served as a platform for Luce's own vision of China, UCR leadership consciously shaped the image of China they sought to promote. As noted by Jespersen, "Although it never operated from overtly political motives as Time Inc. did, the agency nonetheless furthered the same false impressions about China as a land very much like the U.S.; that is, the Chinese people held the same ideals as Americans, and they sought to replace their ancient and outmoded past with a more workable future closely based upon the American example."[39] The distinction was raised that this was not something forced upon the Chinese by foreigners, but invited by them. As Luce once commented on American educational institutions in China, "If this is imperialism . . . the Chinese would say: of this imperialism send us and give us more and more."[40] While Luce's assessment on the reception of American education in China may be debated, he consistently spoke of the Chinese with great respect.

Like AMBASD publicity of its work in Spain, UCR offered a portrait of the Chinese recipients of American relief as sharing a common religious and political heritage. As Jesperson has argued, "Because many of its participating agencies were religiously affiliated, UCR functioned, at least in part, as a missionary organization," which "meant that the Chinese people's acceptance of Christianity" consistently appeared in UCR material.[41] At the same time, portraying China as a nation with a long democratic tradition became a second priority. Given the realities of China's recent political history, this argument was promoted more in social, rather than political, terms. UCR depicted the U.S. and China as allies in the war effort, well before America officially entered the war. As Garside argued, "Help to China means that she can win a fight which is as much ours as hers," in which "the Chinese people are holding the Western ramparts for us . . . for the democratic way of life in the world."[42] Helping China helped American interests, for "a free and independent China will turn to us for all the products that American industry and mechanical genius can produce," guiding both nations "to new heights of prosperity."[43]

UCR's fundraising activities varied. There were Chinese markets, selling tea and other imported goods to raise money. There were radio broadcasts and speaker events. After visiting China themselves in the spring of 1941, Luce and his wife, Clare Booth Luce, returned to report on their travels at a fundraising dinner at the Waldorf-Astoria. Annual Christmas card sales were popular, combining, according to Jespersen, the twin historical roots of American interest in China—Christianity and capitalism.[44] Board member David O. Selznick helped arrange the auction of a number of original Hollywood manuscripts, including that of *Gone with the Wind*. Luce himself wrote a direct appeal to the subscribers of *Time* in the fall of 1941. In the end, UCR fell short of its first $5 million goal, raising only $3.25 million. However, this figure was still significantly higher than the total raised by its separate member agencies in the year prior.[45] Even with such financial advantages, however, some member agencies still chafed with UCR control.

While offering benefits, the centralization of power under UCR challenged the organizational identities of many of its member agencies. The ABMAC had prided itself on arguably being able to respond more rapidly to urgent needs, unburdened by a large bureaucratic apparatus. Prior to incorporation under UCR, agencies had complete freedom in defining their own activities and policies. When a survey by the Rockefeller group reportedly advised that the CAC and the ABMAC disband completely to become a part of the united effort, the suggestion was "met with such a furore [sic] from the Agencies that it could not be put across."[46] However, the "logic of centralization" eventually triumphed, although the ABMAC remained perhaps the most resistant of UCR's constituent agencies to join the coordinated effort. It had only agreed to join UCR with the understanding that UCR would act solely in a financial capacity, leaving the ABMAC free to work with its own contacts in assessing and responding to China's needs.[47]

Despite such formal agreements, UCR staff continued to highlight the intransigence of ABMAC leadership. "Miss Stevens," UCR program director Lennig Sweet wrote, "stands very much on her prerogatives, and will fight at the drop of a hat against anything that seems to be taking away power from

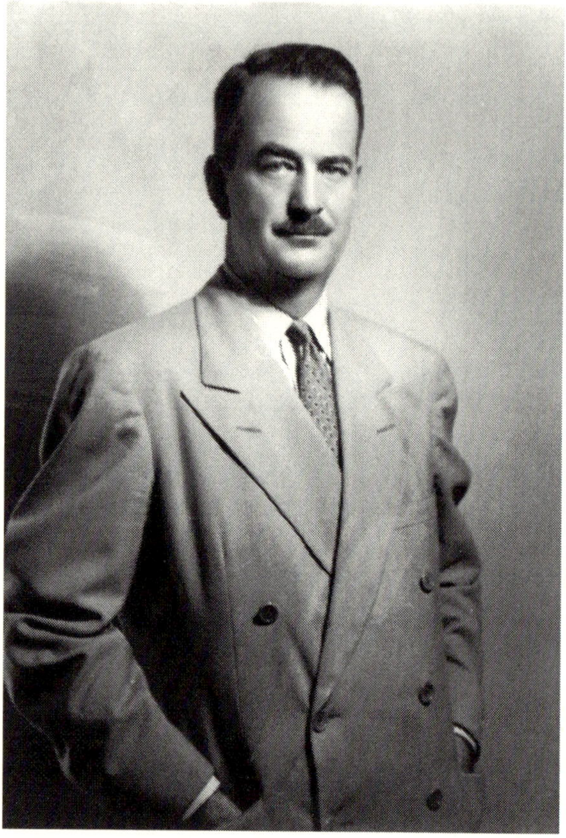

Figure 9. Lennig Sweet of United China Relief (USC Records, Mudd Manuscript Library, Princeton University).

ABMAC" and UCR-ABMAC relations were "not made any easier by the attitude of their leading Chinese doctor [Co Tui], who feels that the Missions are a form of imperialism and that all contacts should be directly with the Chinese."[48]

Many ABMAC leaders saw UCR as dominated by an older generation of Americans, who did not grant Chinese people and institutions the autonomy they were due. Additionally, UCR's efforts to distribute aid more broadly among different Chinese political groups raised other criticisms. For the ABMAC, the Nationalist government led by Chiang Kai-shek was the only legitimate affiliate to be supported in China.

Following their incorporation into a united effort, each member agency of UCR sought to distinguish its work from the others. The ABMAC, from the beginning, sought to establish leadership in medical aid. However, its claims to this field were sometimes challenged by the CAC. The ABMAC further emphasized "its liaison with the Chinese communities in the United States" as well as "its close relationship with the ARC and the China Defense Supplies in [the U.S.] and the Chinese Red Cross and National Health Administration in China."[49]

When the CAC joined UCR, it already had a nationwide network of over fifty local committees. Citing several instances in which it had already begun to coordinate its activities with other agencies, it joined UCR with more enthusiasm than the ABMAC. "We believe," as Chairman Claude Forkner wrote, "that if the coordinating movement is operated on a basis of democratic participation, the various organizations can work together to much better advantage than singly, and that aid to China can be increased many fold over the present amount raised."[50] UCR's greater fundraising potential

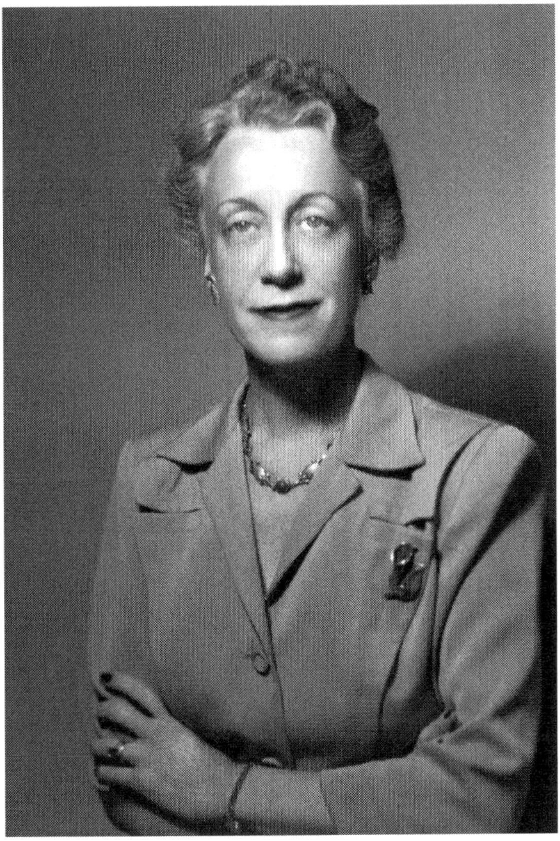

Figure 10. Helen Kennedy Stevens of the American Bureau for Medical Aid to China (USC Records, Mudd Manuscript Library, Princeton University).

overshadowed drawbacks for CAC autonomy. Distinguishing itself from the ABMAC, the CAC noted its activities in the Northwest and close collaboration with the China Defence League as "the only organization assisting the guerrilla areas."[51] In emphasizing the special needs of the Northwest, the CAC noted the region's historic poverty and key strategic location in the Chinese resistance to Japan. The wartime influx of refugees and limited access only compounded the region's pre-existing challenges.

An Alignment of Interests?

Where Spain challenged federal interests in foreign policy, by the time UCR had formed, private aid to China became an opportunity for the state to employ private entities in support of its own interests. However, government regulations still circumscribed private action, and similar restrictions were initially placed on the travel of U.S. citizens to China as had been done on travel to Spain—even before the official outbreak of war in China.[52] Again, exceptions were made for "bona fide newspaper correspondents, bona fide medical workers and persons having urgent and legitimate interests in China."[53]

Since the early 1940s, state structures for managing and overseeing private aid had been steadily expanding. As one contemporary observer noted, while the U.S. "may have been neutral at the time in a military sense . . . there was nothing neutral about the efforts of groups of sympathetic Americans to help sufferers overseas."[54] The State Department continued to require registration for all foreign relief appeals—an action reportedly "not so much to protect American givers from duplicated or unwarranted appeals, but primarily to keep a watchful Federal eye on all matters relating to the countries involved in the war."[55] Within a short period following U.S. entry into World War II, 596 organizations had registered for work in diverse parts of the globe. With private relief appeals multiplying, in 1942 Roosevelt announced the establishment of the President's Committee on War Relief Agencies. Renamed the President's War Relief Control Board a year later, the War Relief Control Board took the registration process out of State Department hands and transferred direct oversight to Roosevelt by requiring the chairman of the board to report to the president.[56] It also meant that the federal government had a role in regulating and coordinating the timing of fundraising events, particularly in light of revived American Red Cross efforts. In other words, it gave the federal government a method of enlisting private charitable enterprise to the broader war effort.

Nominal U.S. involvement in China's fight began well before the official entrance of U.S. forces into the war in December 1941. With the outbreak of war in Europe, the establishment of the Lend-Lease program on 11 March 1941 effectively ended the pretense of American neutrality, eventually promising over $50 billion in aid to Great Britain, the U.S.S.R., France, and China. Although initially designed to offer more direct assistance to Great Britain, Lend-Lease aid was extended to include China in April 1941. Constructed principally with the transfer of war material in mind, small amounts of Lend-Lease aid also trickled through to the medical realm.

The logistics of supplying Lend-Lease funds to Asia was organized primarily through an organization called China Defense Supplies (CDS). Thomas Corcoran, one of Roosevelt's New Deal advisors, officially chartered the organization in Delaware as a civilian corporation. As Corcoran noted, "If we'd tried to set up a government corporation per se, or do the work out of a Federal office there would have been devil to pay on the Hill."[57] In another letter, its purpose was painted slightly differently, as one "organized for the purpose of acting on behalf of the National Government of the Republic of China in respect of securing aid for the Republic of China from the United States of America," in addition to acting as an agent or representative of China in securing Lend-Lease funds.[58] In another document, this one directed to the secretary of state, CDS was described as "designated and . . . acting as an agent, representative, and attorney-in-fact of the Chinese Government, with full power of substitution or delegation, to act either through its own corporate officers or any other corporation or individual designated by it for that purpose."[59] Mutable definitions aside, CDS leadership drew from both American and Chinese representation. Roosevelt's uncle, Frederic Delano (who had spent years in China as a businessman), and T.V. Soong, Chiang's personal representative to Washington, served as co-chairmen.[60] The ABMAC's Co Tui also made regular trips to Washington to advise CDS on medical supplies and coordinate activities with the ARC.[61] In 1944, CDS was reorganized as the China Supplies Commission, with entirely Chinese leadership.[62]

Well before this reorganization, however, attempts to coordinate the activities of relief agencies working in China had been increasing. In 1941, alongside its own return to the scene, the ARC organized a conference on China's medical and public health needs to facilitate an exchange of information about work being done. The meeting's reports, however, were to remain confidential and unreported in the press. Kicking off at ARC headquarters at the end of July, the conference included representatives from a number of organizations and institutions, offering an opportunity for each to begin to define their own spheres of activity within a relief field of increasing complexity.[63] From this conference, it was arranged that the Red Cross would organize civilian relief (and relief of sick and wounded Chinese soldiers, at least where supported by the Chinese Red Cross), while Lend-Lease would offer support to the medical needs of the Chinese Army. Co Tui, representing CDS at the conference, noted that he was in the process of "negotiating to secure medical supplies for the armed forces, armories, and certain defense workers under the Lend-Lease program," working primarily through the Office of Production Management and the War Department. The Lend-Lease administration, he reported, envisaged sixteen aviation hospitals as part of an aviation development program, a medical program for the Yunnan-Burma Railway, and a malaria control project operated by the Public Health Service.[64] Meanwhile, the ABMAC continued to insist that without the "bureaucratic red tape" of these larger institutions, they could still provide more rapid and efficient service for the transmission of medical supplies to both.[65]

The National War Fund

The coalition of private and state efforts being built in the early years of World War II was taken further with the establishment of the National War Fund, announced by Roosevelt in a radio address on 5 October 1943. Although earning the president's support, however, the original impetus does not seem to have come from him. In the words of one of its leaders, the "White House soundingboard" offered an excellent means of introducing the new institution—although its leadership did not specify an alternate source.[66] Drawing from the system of Community Chests (a localized fundraising structure adopted in the aftermath of World War I) the National War Fund's leaders sought to expand the concept of "cooperation through federation" to fundraising on a national level.[67] Community Chest associations were encouraged to form war chests, with more explicit objectives in war relief, and national headquarters set state quotas for fundraising.[68]

The National War Fund provided a federated structure for a diverse array of national relief campaigns, such as UCR. Its stated purposes emphasized the assessment of needs and channeling of resources. However, the National War Fund "could serve no special interest," and "the money contributed . . . had to be disbursed without regard to color, creed, race, or political affiliation"—meaning, for example, that "labor-sponsored projects could not be designed for the relief of labor groups alone, and that no denominational relief program . . . could confine its work to the adherents of its own faith."[69] Such proscriptions ran counter, in many ways, to those of the ABMAC and the CAC. UCR, however, became one of the sixteen original member agencies of the National War Fund, simultaneously yielding some of its fundraising activities to this larger organization. Among other national agencies supported by the National War Fund included American Relief for Italy—and aid was reported as being sent to Germany and Japan as well.[70] However, with National War Fund relief dedicated to the United Seaman's service, United Service Organization (USO) support of American troops, and U.S. prisoners of war, it is difficult to say with certainty how much of this money may have gone to local communities in enemy territory. At least for American Relief for Italy, however, National War Fund promotional materials described support going to civilian victims of the war. It is unknown what kinds of debates may have preceded such action and what kind of controversies may have preceded U.S. aid to enemy territories during and after the war.

Following a model similar to the ARC in its federated structure and largely private financial sourcing guided by state interests, the National War Fund also functioned as a semi-governmental institution. Through the system of locally based war chests, the money it raised did not come from the government itself, but from private citizens making donations to a state-sponsored institution. And the National War Fund insisted upon Washington approval for its projects. A close working relationship with Washington also helped minimize the risk of contributing money to projects for which there was public funding—as "private funds" such as those raised by the National War Fund "should be confined to emergency situations for which no public funds could be found."[71] Meanwhile, the U.S. government found an ally not only in offering support for its own troops (the USO) received substantial support from the National War Fund) and the soldiers and civilians of allied nations, but also in promoting its wartime allegiances to the American public. As summarized by one, "With little or no real authority, and with virtually all its operations dependent on good will, the National War Fund in all its aspects was essentially a public relations operation."[72] In raising money for the allied war effort, the National War Fund had to "sell" the war to the American people.

Meanwhile, the National War Fund's implicit support by the U.S. government gave UCR a degree of formal state recognition that it had long sought. As early as 1941 Luce had written to then secretary of state Cordell Hull seeking a public endorsement from the Roosevelt administration. Hull, however, declined to return the sample (positive) response Luce had enclosed with his letter on the principle that the State Department did not endorse private fundraising organization activities, as a matter of policy. Meanwhile, the federal government's alliances with other private organizations—such as China Defense Supplies or the National War Fund—in situations deemed compatible with state interests suggest that Hull's declination "as a matter of policy" may have been a convenient oversimplification. As cooperation between the government and these ostensibly private agencies increased, so did efforts to define the relative responsibilities of each.

Private vs. Government Action

Working more closely with state enterprise in both the U.S. and China, UCR leadership had to navigate variable expectations of government and private action. Particularly as mediated through the National War Fund, these semi-private institutions fit clearly with historian James Sparrow's "warfare state." The war caused a shift in federal priorities from a focus on preserving national welfare (often at the perceived expense of business subject to greater government regulation) to mobilizing all available resources and manpower for national defense. As described by Sparrow, "Businessmen volunteered to run the war effort at all levels, from local car dealers selling war bonds all the way up to national figures such as Sears, Roebuck President Donald Nelson heading the War Production Board to guide the entire mobilization."[73] The National War Fund's own board of directors reinforces Sparrow's observation of the close affiliation between business leadership and the new war mobilization. This newly constructed relationship between state and private action was largely of mutual benefit. Both parties invoked the imagery and ideology of the "American way" in their work, appealing to patriotically inspired giving as central to the expected participation of the American public. Although private entities, such as UCR, utilized a greater flexibility and responsiveness than might be achieved through strictly governmental channels to their advantage, they simultaneously saw their relationship with federal entities as symbiotic.

The leadership of the National War Fund made an effort to avoid working in areas where public funds were available. As private efforts, they defined their contribution to the U.S. war effort in filling in gaps left by the government. But implicit in the activities of the National War Fund (and UCR) was the expectation that the U.S. government should be doing something to help foreign populations such as the Chinese. For the members of UCR, this expectation existed before any formal alliance existed between China and the U.S.; in the case of the National War Fund, such expectations developed with America's formal wartime definitions of "friend" and "foe." At the same time, in cooperating with Chinese agencies, UCR also held expectations of the role of the Chinese government. In fact, UCR officials saw their work as serving as an impetus for greater government action. In 1943, Edwards reported that "it has been practically assured that the government grant 50 cents on a dollar for our projects and dollar for dollar on direct relief work," going on to argue that "certainly they should match the program more than dollar for dollar."[74] At least for Edwards, American aid came with the expectation that the Chinese government would contribute equally.

The question of private versus state funding responsibility seems to have become particularly heated in regard to the Emergency Medical Services Training Schools (EMSTS). With support for the program split between the Chinese Red Cross and Army Medical Administration, EMSTS funding was complex, without considering the addition of outside funds from the ABMAC and UCR. The controversy over Lim's leadership exacerbated matters.[75] Edwards argued that as a "government project" the EMSTS "should be entirely under government support" and UCR "will be quite within its rights as donors to withhold support of government operations, in which there is small or practically no government financial support."[76] ABMAC leadership, however, continued to see Lim's EMSTS as one of the most important projects on their budget.

Following the military alliance between the U.S. and China, the ABMAC increasingly prioritized military medical support within its general emphasis on assisting Nationalist forces. Restating its objectives in a policy statement in 1944, the ABMAC clearly delineated its first priority as supporting the "medical effort directed toward the successful prosecution of total war" while pursuing the secondary objective of promoting "the development of wartime medical projects which will have continued usefulness after the war."[77] In other words, military needs were to supersede those of civilians. ABMAC aid sent to military medical services increased in 1943 and 1944, with nearly half of its funds directed toward the Army Medical Administration and the Chinese Red Cross.[78] Three quarters of this budget went to training, with the rest dedicated to supporting preventive medical and surgical units working in the field. In making recommendations for UCR's medical budget, the medical committee formed by the ABMAC proposed, "60% of the medical appropriations go to the Army Medical Service and 30% to the Civilian Medical

Service and 9% to medical education."[79] When UCR's Committee on Coordination (led by Edwards in Chungking) overrode this recommendation, the decision led to a major rift in ABMAC-UCR relations. In ABMAC president Donald D. Van Slyke's view, the coordination committee's decision wrongly short changed support of China's military medical services. UCR, meanwhile, claimed such a division of funds had "no rational basis whatever" and overlapped unnecessarily with their expectation that Lend-Lease funds were to cover any needed foreign support of China's military. More fundamentally, UCR and ABMAC leadership seemed to disagree on expectations of state responsibility.

ABMAC frustration at the perceived limits imposed by UCR on its action also contributed to the deterioration of the relationship between the two organizations. ABMAC leadership blamed UCR for stifling the initiative and action of participating agencies. These limitations arose most prominently relevant to ABMAC engagement with Chinese government and military institutions. The ABMAC's attempt to break away from UCR and establish a relationship directly under the president's War Relief Control Board as an independent group was denied. By the board's assessment, while "they did not wish to force a merger, they had made UCR responsible for the distributing and the raising of relief funds in China" and the ABMAC must, therefore, remain under UCR.[80] The entrance of the National War Fund exacerbated the problem for the ABMAC. "So long as the US public, through the National War Fund, supplies funds," one ABMAC report concluded, "UCR bids fair to eliminate or emasculate the Participating Agencies and become the US Almoner to poor China, forgetting the purpose of the donors, and their own code of obligation to fighting men engaged in a critical and supreme struggle against the common aggressor."[81] The ABMAC charged UCR with failing to provide sufficient assistance to the Chinese soldier and the underlying conflict, which they saw as the source for the "misery and want" UCR sought to address.[82] The ABMAC seemed to use USO service to the American soldier as the standard for what UCR should be giving to the Chinese soldier, arguing that the National War Fund already supplied more than half of its funds to the USO.

Civilian and Military Tensions

The U.S. government's interest in the humanitarian medical relief practiced by UCR and its member agencies went beyond assistance to the civilian victims of war—although these were often the recipients highlighted in UCR publicity. State interest in UCR efforts was an interest in aid as an extension of military enterprise, both as a logistical method to maintain sufficient manpower, and as a way to encourage sympathies between the U.S. and China. As Far East advisor Lauchlin Currie advised to President Roosevelt in March 1941, "One of the most effective ways of encouraging China and deterring Japan would be to go out of our way in giving evidences of friendship, close collaboration and admiration for China," a mission that "can be done both overtly and through 'inspired' stories coming out of Washington."[83] Support of humanitarian aid initiatives fit neatly with Currie's advice.

UCR and its member organizations, however, often varied in their own interpretation. In 1945, for instance, the Chinese government offered UCR office space from which to work. However, UCR's Lennig Sweet declined this offer, noting that since "UCR is not a military or diplomatic organization . . . we feel that it would not be justified or wise for us to make use of the kind offices of the Chinese government to provide us with quarters under the regulations for the requisitioning of property."[84] Yet others within UCR had connections that fell outside of Sweet's assessment. The volunteers of the ABMAC blood bank, for instance, all received a commission in the Chinese army before their departure from the U.S. By this time, the U.S. and China had become formal military allies, creating a very different set of circumstances for the American volunteers that did make it to China.

In contrast, the similarly murky status of AMBASD volunteers in Spain caused significant controversy for the organization. Although the medical volunteers sent to Spain by the AMBASD essentially became part of the Republican military medical services, through the International Brigades, the organization simultaneously cited the standards of neutrality touted by the Red Cross. The reality on the ground was not always so clear. As ambulance driver James Neugass wrote, "Since I do not wish to exaggerate the fashion in which Rebel wounded are treated by the People's Army, I must state that we bring in our wounded before we risk our lives carrying Theirs."[85] But when "Their" wounded were attended to, treating the enemy patient had the purpose both of curing the wounds inflicted by the war—and also in "converting" him politically.[86]

Neugass, as an ambulance driver in Spain, wavered in identifying himself as part of the military or as something separate from it. Within the first ten pages of his memoir, Neugass wrote of being part of a "we" consisting of "the best semi-professional army," which also "hated death and war and . . . could never manage to think of ourselves precisely as soldiers." Neugass demonstrated an affection and affiliation with the military forces of the International Brigades, while also feeling separate and alienated from it. Later, disgusted by the use of Republican ambulances as military targets, Neugass wrote: "I've been an instinctive pacifist and a hater of flags and uniforms and, above all, martial music all my life; but I feel that if I catch the man who rolls rocks onto the Mas de las Matas road, I'd like to open him up little by little with my jackknife until I see if I can tell a fascist heart from a democratic heart."[87] Neugass's words demonstrate not only the transformative experience of being immersed in a zone of conflict, but also the blurry space occupied by AMBASD personnel, particularly the ambulance drivers whose work often brought them into the heart of the battle. And it was this uncertain role that had become a question of concern for the U.S. State Department. Examining the political debate at home alongside the experience of the individuals who traveled to Spain and China as representatives and volunteers offers a compelling and valuable contrast.

Conclusions

The period discussed in this chapter highlights where trajectories in the development of private aid to Spain and China began to differ. From 1939, the Spanish Civil War and Second Sino-Japanese War were clearly headed in different directions, and the American organizations discussed here paralleled those developments. As the AMBASD faded, the ABMAC and the CAC picked up momentum through the newly founded UCR. On one level, this waxing and waning of influence may be interpreted on the changing needs of the targeted recipients and the variations in organization publicity. But the relationships of these organizations with the U.S. government also became important: where UCR found its interests allied with the federal government, the AMBASD remained at odds with State Department policy.

In these developing alliances, however, neither the state nor the private activists discussed can be described as being the sole drivers of change. Certainly, in terms of overall influence and resources available, federal policies and institutions did have an upper hand. However, private groups were still able to organize significant programs of aid outside of government policy. Meanwhile, other factors, such as cultural or racial sympathies or prejudices seemed to have limited influence on ultimate success. The Spanish, for instance, shared a common Western culture and heritage with the U.S., whereas the Chinese still faced significant legal prejudices in the U.S. as organizations such as the ABMAC first began. However, instead of dictating success for

Spanish aid and failure for Chinese aid, the establishment of organizations such as UCR actually contributed to major shifts in American state and public attitudes toward Chinese-Americans. While the issue of whether efforts fell under a civilian or military category was highlighted in debates, the larger political overtones ultimately seem to have taken precedent. Where the State Department found allegiance with organizations sending aid to China with China's rising role as a military ally, it never resolved its tensions over the activities of the roughly 150 Americans who traveled to Spain under the auspices of the AMBASD.

CHAPTER FOUR

American Medical Volunteers In Spain

The first unit of American medical volunteers set out for Spain in January 1937. A few months later, the passage of the Neutrality Act of 1937 expanded previous legislation seeking to limit and define U.S. participation in foreign conflicts. While explicit in prohibiting the export of any arms and other war materiel to belligerent nations, the Neutrality Acts were less explicit in circumscribing citizen action. In 1935, U.S. citizens had been warned that travel to war zones would be done at their own risk. In 1937, U.S. citizens were explicitly forbidden from traveling on the ships of belligerent nations. The reportedly humanitarian activities of the AMBASD did not fall neatly into any category, despite the State Department's efforts to define them more clearly.

The nearly 150 American medical volunteers sent by the AMBASD to join the medical services Republican military forces and the International Brigades did so with the permission of the U.S. government, their passports marked "valid for Spain." But this permission had only come after a letter-writing campaign by the AMBASD and small public outcry to reverse an earlier prohibition on travel. For some volunteers, this special permission to contribute to Republican Spain was a motivation in and of itself. For many more, the motivations and rationale behind volunteering with the AMBASD were complex. Although few cite defiance of U.S. policy as an explicit goal, many reported on feeling the need to go to Spain because there wasn't enough being done from other sources. While AMBASD leadership encouraged a proactive stance in promoting the cause of the Second Spanish Republic, AMBASD volunteers were generally immersed in a different reality and different set of concerns once they arrived in Spain. Their physical presence in Spain offered an opportunity to witness the conflict firsthand and report home on what they saw. The role of witness sought to inspire both greater political and humanitarian action, reinforcing the intertwined influences in the organization's identity. In many ways, the work of AMBASD volunteers came to define the organization itself.

Republican Military Medical Services

The AMBASD's first unit set sail from New York City on 16 January 1937 with varied expectations over where exactly their units would serve. Nurse Fredericka Martin described leaving with a "semi-romantic notion of attaching themselves to Spanish [army] units" in the same way that "foreign ambulance units had worked with French outfits in World War I."[1] Meanwhile, Barsky envisioned "help from America in such quantities" and "so closely identified with the Loyalist forces" that it "would be impossible to distinguish between the two."[2] Although the group's organizers had been in contact with representatives of the Republican government, their understanding of what they would find in Spain still seemed fairly vague. Their first assumptions, based on reports suggesting that the Republican government had no medical service of its own, were relatively accurate. Republican Spain had suddenly lost most of its military medical services with the army's rebellion in July, leaving the civilian medical community with the daunting task of recreating a new military medical service.[3] Nevertheless, during the first months of war, efforts to expand the Republic's medical services were carried out "with almost excessive enthusiasm" as hospitals were founded by political parties, trade unions, and almost any group whose leaders were inspired by enough "fantasy, generosity, and a greater or lesser degree of expertise."[4] By the end of 1936, a medical service of some six hundred doctors (of whom only one hundred or so had military experience) had developed.[5]

Others seemed to have had the impression that the American unit would become part of ICRC medical services. As Barsky stated plainly in his memoir, "We had been told in New York—or perhaps 'commanded' is the word—to ally ourselves with the International Red Cross in Spain."[6] The Red Cross, they were told, had assumed the responsibility of organizing the collaborative efforts of "other similarly medical-minded people" from around the world. A Red Cross hospital had supposedly been set up in Madrid with the various national groups of volunteers operating as independent divisions within the hospital. Barsky continued, "I think most of us even had some sort of mental picture of the building itself and saw the kindly efficient personnel going about their business, yet not too busy to welcome the newly arrived American outfit."[7] Upon reaching Madrid, however, the unit found no such hospital.

While the ICRC may have been largely absent from Spanish soil, the Spanish Red Cross in Madrid was not. By the time the American unit arrived, over thirty hospitals were functioning in Madrid, at least two of which seem to have been Spanish Red Cross facilities.[8] The Spanish Red Cross was particularly busy in the first months of the conflict. Working along the Madrid front, and later expanding into the fronts of Andalucía, Extremadura, and Levante, Spanish Red Cross personnel recovered wounded from the front lines, evacuating them to first aid points and field hospitals established by the Red Cross.[9]

Whatever their initial vision had been—adjunct to the Spanish army or auxiliary to the Red Cross—the leaders of the AMBASD's first unit had to reassess their role upon arrival. "The only thing we heard about that bore a faint resemblance to this ideal conception," Barsky claimed, "was the Hospital No.1 run by the Internationals in Albacete."[10] Barsky, Martin, and administrative assistant and translator Mildred Rackley split off from the rest of the group to determine where to direct AMBASD resources. The advice they received was the same everywhere: for "linguistic and logistic reasons" they should join the medical services of the International Brigades. Although Rackley served as a translator, she seemed to be one of the few with Spanish language skills. Even Spanish and English combined were not necessarily enough for the incredibly multilingual International Brigades, which at times became "a veritable tower of Babel."[11]

While working alongside the Spanish Republican army had been a part of the group's earliest plans, they seemed hesitant about affiliating with the International Brigades. On the ship from New York, Barsky talked of needing to ensure that AMBASD volunteers did not "openly fraternize" with the ninety or so young men aboard rumored to be enlisting in Lincoln-Washington Brigade.[12] With the association of the International Brigades with the Communist Party, Barsky suggested that such affiliations could seriously limit the AMBASD's support at home. Meanwhile, Martin argued that the group's hesitation to associate with the International Brigades stemmed less from political concerns and more simply from the fact that "U.S. volunteers had come out of admiration for the Spanish people and wanted to work directly with them."[13] Even after agreeing to join the International Brigade medical services, the Americans insisted on maintaining a high degree of autonomy. Although "the Estado Major and the chiefs of the Medical Service of the International Brigade considered the American request naïve and ridiculous," the request was eventually granted.[14]

The Medical Services of the International Brigades

The first unit's arrival in Spain was almost perfectly timed with the establishment of the International Brigades' own medical services. That same month, Dr. Oskar Telge, a Bulgarian, had been appointed director of the *Servicio*

Sanitario Internacional (SSI) and given the task of organizing the medical services of the International Brigades.[15] Originally, neither the Republican military nor the International Brigades saw the need to create separate medical services for the international forces. However, Spain's international volunteers posed a much greater challenge than had been expected. Dispersed among various hospitals, wounded internationals became easily isolated.[16] Creating a separate medical service for the International Brigades sought to provide a solution for both "linguistic and logistic" problems.

Many international volunteers seemed to appreciate the new organizational structure. Although most wounded Americans writing home from Spain's hospitals and convalescent centers spoke highly of the medical services as a whole, many letters home show an increasing dissatisfaction with the care provided in Spanish or other international hospitals as the writers waited expectantly to be transferred to an American facility.[17] Even in a group with such an internationalist outlook as the International Brigades, the strains and stresses of injury and illness seemed enough to make the most open-minded patient dream fondly of the comforts and traditions of home. American hospitals provided medical staff with familiar understandings of health and illness, as well as familiar food, which was often cited as better than the more typically Spanish fare of other hospitals. Favorite holidays, such as Halloween, Thanksgiving, and Christmas, could also be celebrated in ways that reminded American volunteers of home.

Carl Geiser's correspondence home between October 1937 and January 1938 illustrates the pleasures and frustrations of being a patient in this international climate. Born in Ohio and a member of the Young Communist League from the early 1930s, Geiser left for Spain to join the International Brigades in April 1937. Although Geiser's first observation after being wounded at Fuentes de Ebro was of the "excellence" of Spain's medical services, his positive attitude degenerated as his expected transfer to an American hospital was delayed for weeks.[18] Geiser referred repeatedly to the isolation he felt as being one of few—and sometimes the only—Americans in the hospital to which he was confined. Geiser frequently discussed the strange and frustrating customs he observed in Spanish hospitals: the provision of wine instead of water as a bedside beverage, and the Spanish doctors' persistent inability to cure his diarrhea—a common complaint among foreigners in Spain. Even the poor sweeping technique of a Spanish nurse was noted as proof of the country's "backwardness."[19] He summed up his frustration in one letter: "I am furious over being left here when I know I would receive better treatment at Benicasim."[20] As another wounded American admitted simply in a letter home, after a series of letters commending the care and facilities of the American hospital where he was stationed, "I pour out my grief in letters . . . because I'm cranky and grouchy about being laid up so long—and since I restrain myself from it here I try to take it out on the people I write to."[21]

The establishment of the SSI was supported by the parallel creation of the *Centrale Sanitaire Internacionale* (CSI) in Paris. The CSI's development was largely due to the efforts of French physician Pierre Roqués.[22] Roqués had been working in Spain since October 1936, along with a handful of other foreign doctors who became the foundation of the International Brigade medical services.[23] Roqués's efforts were further aided by the Comintern, which supported the CSI and used it as the primary conduit for donations of medical supplies and personnel.[24] The CSI also became the umbrella organization for directing the deployment of volunteer medical personnel and donated material from dozens of different countries.

It is unclear exactly how much communication existed between the AMBASD and the CSI. In April 1937, Barsky referred to coordination and purchasing committees for the Sanitary Service of the International Brigade having been set up in Paris under the leadership of Dr. Roqués. He noted that he would "attempt to establish connections" with Roqués as quickly as possible, although he also noted that these committees were "not functioning as well as they should be."[25] Later in the war, San Francisco surgeon Leo Eloesser seemed largely ignorant of the CSI's role and activities. Writing to an American colleague at home, he wondered exactly what the CSI's duties were and who was in charge of its operation and staffing, both in Spain and in Paris. "Both places are slip shod and inefficient," Eloesser continued, and "I can cite many instances of delay and neglect in both offices."[26] Still, letters between the CSI in Paris and AMBASD in New York show there was some communication between the two organizations, even if AMBASD doctors in the field had relatively low awareness or opinions of its work.

By the fall of 1937, the SSI counted in its ranks nearly two hundred fifty doctors, five hundred nurses or orderlies, and over six hundred stretcher-bearers of more than twenty different nationalities.[27] The Spanish formed the largest group, followed by American, English, German, and Polish volunteers. Between January 1937 and November 1938, the AMBASD sent more than a dozen units of volunteers to Spain. By the middle of 1938, these volunteers were involved (in varying degrees) in running eight hospitals, while up to three American surgical teams were traveling the front lines in mobile operating units at any given time.[28] The extent of the Americans' resources may have even become a source of some discord within the international services. While Spanish publicity at their arrival warmly welcomed the new volunteers, some noted that it also "raised contrary feelings in Internationals toiling in hospitals with not even rags enough for bandages."[29] Beyond recognition for reportedly being the largest and most well equipped of the national units in Spain, Barsky himself took on a leadership role as director of all foreign aid units when the SSI was reorganized under the aegis of the *Inspección General*.[30]

The SSI also reportedly attracted its share of "*aventureros y falsarios*."[31] And many more of those with the best of intentions simply lacked experience in the reality and practice of war medicine. As summarized by historian Nicolas Coni, "Although some of the surgical teams were excellent, many left something to be desired, and there was a resentful feeling especially among some of their Spanish colleagues that they had come to learn by practising on the wounded as if they had arrived in a third-world country."[32] American nurse Mary Platkin remembered the disparity between her own expectations and the reality she encountered upon her arrival at the hospital at Benicasim. As she confessed to her diary, "I found out very quickly that with all the intrigues between the various nationalities, the undercurrent of opportunists, etc. that everything was just a little different. That although we're all fighting for one grand cause, there was entirely too much petty rot going on between the various groups giving me the impression that each was seeking glory, glory, and more glory."[33]

The contributions of national relief committees, facilitated by the CSI, formed the SSI's basis of support. American contributions constituted the largest portion, giving over 900,000 francs over the course of the war.[34] Donations from national relief societies were supplemented by support from the army's medical service and the *Socorro Rojo Internacional*, in addition to donations from the brigaders themselves.[35] At its peak in 1937, the SSI boasted over five thousand hospital beds in over thirty different hospitals supported by a central pharmacy, a fleet of ambulances and *auto-chirs* (mobile operating rooms), departments of chemical defense and hygiene and disinfection, and a school for training nursing orderlies.[36]

Although it was officially subject to the Republican Ministry of War, the SSI maintained significant autonomy in running the medical services for the International Brigades over its first year of existence. Coni notes that doctors and nurses working in its service were "only very transiently" given uniforms or military ranks.[37] While this may have been true in the earliest days of the war, as the conflict progressed—and particularly after the international sanitary service was reorganized under Republican military medical services—military rank played an increasingly prominent role. International medical volunteers were given a *carnet militar,* which included a photo, basic biographical data, profession, and political affiliation.[38] Although the International Brigades may have presented itself as a new type of more democratic fighting force—and indeed some militias strove to maintain social equity between officers and men—military hierarchies still held an important place in practice. Martin suggested that citing military rank could be crucial in providing treatment to the "reluctant, scared, or obstinate patient" who would "haggle he did not need to obey" if the nurse or technician was of a lower rank.[39] At the same time, Martin lamented the fact that too many—"even among our U.S. doctors"—were "childish" in their desire to get "the highest number of stripes going." Nevertheless, she concluded that "on the whole we internationals, from the States and England especially, although in uniform . . . lived and worked exactly as if we were not under military orders. We merely in thought and deed cooperated with the military in order to take care of the wounded and assumed we were equally responsible for the civilian sick around us as we were for civilian wounded in air raids."[40]

While it operated relatively independently of the Republican army's sanitary service, the SSI followed a similar model structurally—a structure informed by precedents set during World War I. A branching hierarchy of medical stations and hospitals developed, extending from the front lines to the rear. Orderlies and stretcher-bearers staffed first aid posts assigned to companies along the front. Where possible, each battalion within the International Brigades had a medical officer of its own nationality.[41] Mobile surgical teams operated near the front lines, supported by ambulances and *auto-chirs.* By the end of 1937, three Spanish, two Catalan, three American, and two British surgical teams were working at the front in this capacity.[42] Field hospitals provided the next line of assistance, with services for internal medicine and venereal disease. These hospitals were set up to convert easily to entirely surgical hospitals should battle conditions lead to a particularly high influx of wounded. Moving further along the route of evacuation, rearguard hospitals provided care for less urgent injuries. The International Brigade's major base hospitals were established in the town of Huete, near Madrid; at Benicasim, north of Valencia along the Mediterranean coast; and at La Pasionara Hospital in Murcia.[43] Convalescent centers provided support for more long-term recoveries. All International Brigade hospitals were open to both brigaders and Spanish patients, with civilians receiving treatment at many of them as well.[44] American physician Irving Busch reported in 1938 that of all the wounded treated by U.S. volunteers in Spain, 80 percent were Spanish and the remaining 20 percent "internationals."[45]

As the war progressed, the parallel structures of the SSI and Republican *Inspección General de Sanidad* grew closer. By the end of January 1938, the SSI became a subsection of the *Inspección General* under the new name of *Ayuda Médica Extranjera.* With the SSI's director operating under the orders of the *Inspección*, the SSI's headquarters were relocated from Albacete to the *Inspección*'s office in Barcelona.[46] Meanwhile, donations processed by the CSI specifically for the International Brigades could continue to be directed to international volunteers. The CSI's Paris office formally recognized the reorganization in March 1938.[47] As the CSI advised AMBASD headquarters in April 1938, "For the future, you should not use propaganda which speaks of six American hospitals in Spain, for the situation is now entirely changed" and "propaganda should now stress the needs for the Spanish Sanitary Service, to which the foreign services are attached under the direction of Dr. Barsky."[48] However, the newly reorganized medical services lasted less than a year before all international volunteers—including those in the medical services—were asked to leave Spain by Prime Minister Juan Negrín, who hoped to appeal to the Western democracies by ejecting all foreign involvement in the Republican forces.

The First Three Months: From Romeral to Villa Paz

After meeting with leaders of the International Brigades and their medical services in Albacete, the first unit traveled to the small town of Romeral south of Madrid. After consulting with the village *alcalde*, the group moved into a recently built schoolhouse, unloading twenty tons of hospital supplies within the next two days.[49] In unpacking, the group discovered that five boxes of material had disappeared in transit, including the group's two sterilizers—essential for any surgical activity. Mildred Rackley and driver Carl Rahman went out in search of a replacement and found a discarded one at a nearby hospital, which Rahman was able to repair to basic function—although it left clothes and instruments wet from the steaming process. Numerous other logistical problems had to be overcome in the weeks that followed. Organizing food, water, and electricity all proved major challenges. As Barsky recalled later, "Already money was of no value and food the precious thing."[50] Spain's food shortage only became worse as the war continued.[51] Meanwhile, electricity in the village was unreliable and was switched off entirely whenever enemy aircraft flew over the sector.[52] Stories of the completion of operations by flashlight or candlelight became a common motif in reports to AMBASD headquarters in New York and volunteers' letters home.

As the lines of battle shifted, AMBASD volunteers soon received orders to move. The unit had arrived at the height of the Battle of Jarama—a Nationalist drive to take over Madrid that was ultimately rebuffed, albeit at a high human cost for both sides. Less than six weeks after their arrival in Romeral, the majority of the first unit found themselves in Tarancón.[53] Northwest of Romeral on the road from Madrid to Valencia, Tarancón was established as an evacuation point for wounded with three small hospitals. The hospitals, however, seriously lacked equipment and staff. When the Americans arrived they found only a few beds and a Spanish surgical team with no instruments.[54]

Following their relative independence in Romeral, the Americans were frustrated by the situation in Tarancón. Almost immediately upon their arrival, "everybody was giving orders" as American equipment and ambulances were dispersed.[55] "We soon found it was going to be a pretty mixed up American Hospital," Rackley recalled, and "Eddie concluded that the only reason they had wanted us to come to Tarancón was to get hold of our equipment."[56] The confusion of Tarancón seems to have been exacerbated by conflicts higher in the chain of command, with two different officials giving Barsky orders. It was decided that the American unit would move out of Tarancón and establish a base hospital nearby, where they would have greater autonomy. A handful of American personnel worked in Tarancón on and off throughout the remaining year, until the hospitals were largely destroyed in heavy bombing in December 1937.[57]

In early April, the Americans—joined by a second and third unit from the states—moved on to the nearby town of Saelices, where they set up a new hospital (Villa Paz) and convalescent centre (Castillejo). The hospitals occupied one of the favored summer homes of the Spanish royal family and were still filled with antique furniture, fine art, and a library full of richly bound books. Lofted granaries became wards, the stable a dining room, and the servants' quarters staff accommodation. A stream ran through the valley, with a dam to generate electric power. There were gardens at each hospital, cultivated by patients and staff.[58] Over the following summer, the staff at Villa Paz dealt with over 2,500 admissions of wounded during the Battle of Brunete.[59] Villa Paz also received visits from two American congressmen.[60]

While Villa Paz remained the main American hospital center throughout the war, U.S. volunteers worked at a number of other hospitals throughout

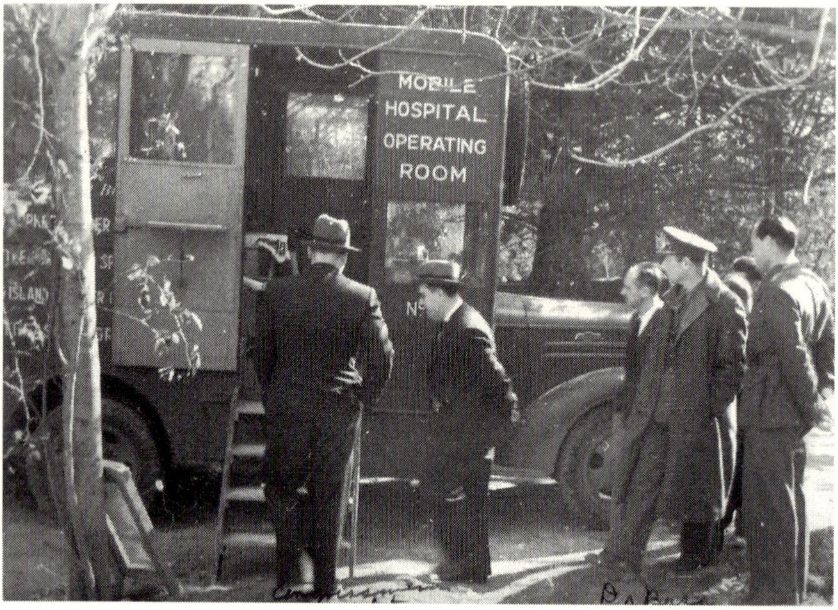

Figure 11. Congressmen Bernard and O'Connell visiting AMBASD units in Spain (Barsky Photograph Collection, Tamiment Library, New York University).

Spain. The convalescent center at Benicasim was one of these. As described by an American patient, "The place I am staying at is beautiful, one doesn't even know that there is a war going on in this part of Spain . . . Imagine me living in a villa with marble floors and stairs, furnished with antique Spanish furniture, with the inner garden known as the patio or courtyard full of statues and fountains and huge luscious grapes hanging down from overhead vines, surrounded by orange and lemon trees."[61] Nurse and physical therapist Luba Brisker helped set up the Benicasim's physical therapy department before going on to do the same in Mataró in Catalonia.[62] The three hospitals of Murcia all had American personnel on their staff, with Dr. Frances Vanzant in charge of a hospital for internal diseases and Dr. Sidney Vogel in charge of a surgical hospital.[63] Meanwhile, a number of smaller hospitals were set up or maintained by American personnel along the front lines of battle.

The Mobile Units: Along the Córdoba, Teruel, and Aragon Fronts

As the Americans settled into Villa Paz and Castillejo, plans were being made to send a unit to the south. Led by Barsky, thirty-four AMBASD volunteers

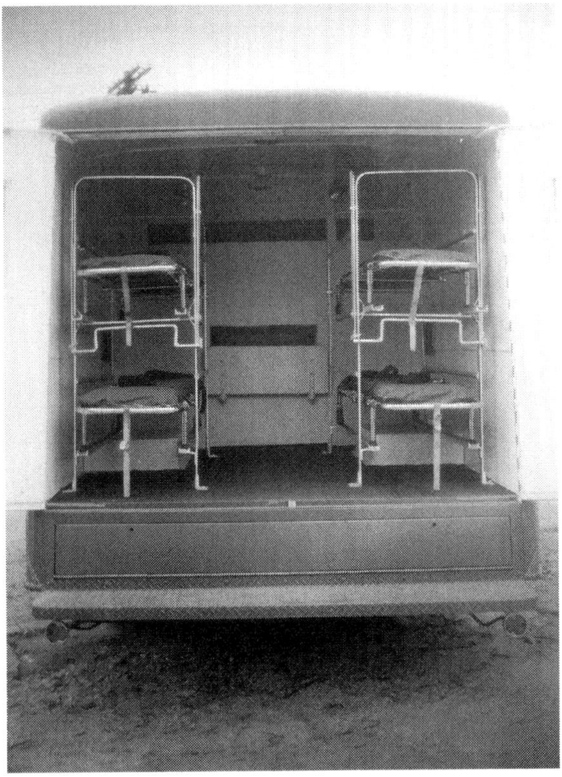

Figure 12. An AMBASD ambulance: an important tool for mobile units (Barsky Photograph Collection, Tamiment Library, New York University).

traveled to the Córdoba front, where they established front-line hospitals in Pozoblanco and Belalcazar and worked as a mobile surgical unit traveling the front lines in an *auto-chir.*[64] Introduced during World War I, use of the *auto-chir* and mobile operating teams was vastly expanded in the Spanish Civil War.[65] By enabling surgeons to operate much nearer to the front, transport time for critically injured patients could be greatly reduced.

At the front, enemy artillery and aviation became a much more immediate reality for the medical services, which often had to operate under fire. Infectious diseases such as malaria and dysentery were also endemic in much of the Spanish south, and AMBASD volunteers found themselves treating large numbers of both combatants and civilians for these diseases.[66] Chief of Belalcazar, Dr. Norman Rintz, who reportedly picked up "the malaria bug" himself, established a separate malaria ward to meet demand.[67] American volunteers worked along the Córdoba front throughout the summer, celebrating the Fourth of July in the mobile hospital with members of the

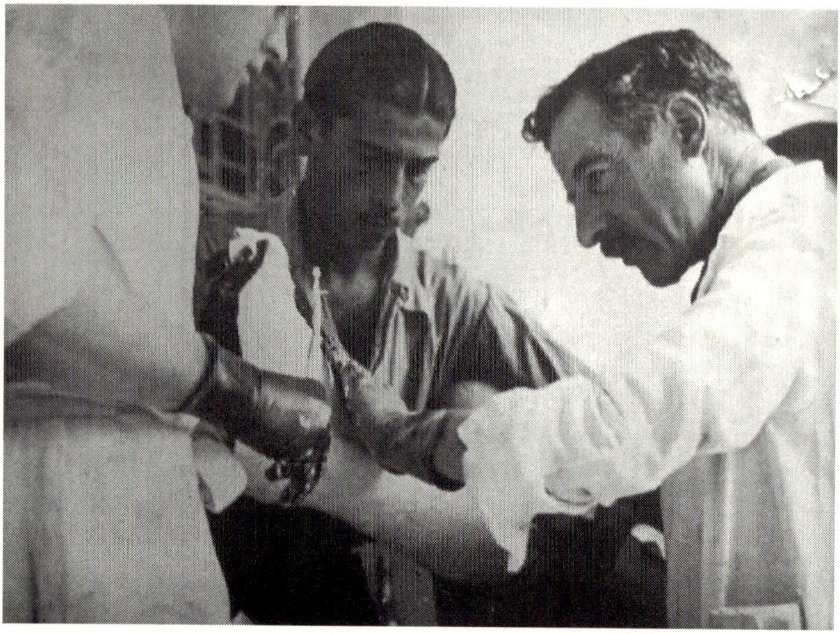

Figure 13. Eloesser (right) at work in Spain (Martin Photograph Collection, Tamiment Library, New York University).

13th International Brigade and 86th Spanish Brigade.[68] Eventually all staff returned to Villa Paz when the southern hospitals were evacuated in early November of 1937. That autumn, Barsky returned from the U.S. with a new unit, including San Francisco surgeon Leo Eloesser, surgeon Edwin Sherman Weisfield of Seattle, nurse Ave Bruzzichesi of New Jersey, and several ambulance drivers, including the writer James Neugass.[69]

The following winter, American mobile units moved north to the Teruel front. While the summer in southern Spain had been oppressively hot, both Republican and Nationalist forces had to fight frigid temperatures and snow in the mountains of Teruel. As described by Neugass, Teruel became "Valley Forge and Verdun and the North Pole combined."[70] A group of American volunteers, again led by Barsky, arrived at their first base just before Christmas. They spent New Year's Eve pushing a convoy of ambulances and support vehicles up steep mountain roads through a blizzard that had forced nearly all fighting to a temporary standstill.[71] A unit of West Coast volunteers, led by Eloesser, also traveled to the Teruel front, establishing a two-hundred–bed hospital in Alfambra.[72] In the spring of 1937, Barsky led yet another mobile surgical team, this time to the Aragon front. He was not there long, however, before being called to Barcelona to take over the newly reorganized international medical services. By this time, Barsky himself seems to have been showing signs of fatigue. As described by Neugass: "Major B's health is bad . . . Nothing but our bread suits his ulcerated stomach, and nothing but cigarettes will ease his nerves. Tobacco hurts his stomach more than the oranges he eats after he stops the car and throws up what he has mistakenly eaten . . . His nerves and sensitivity and introspection are not those of the soldier [that] will-power and political convictions have made."[73] Spain certainly tested the convictions of U.S. volunteers, affecting more than Barsky alone. By mid-February, Neugass reported medical staff numbers to have fallen from thirty-two to seventeen.[74] As Republican forces were forced back in the Ebro Retreat, Barsky's mobile unit scrambled to keep up with the casualties and constant movement. Remarkably, up through that February, none of the medical volunteers of Barksy's unit had been wounded.

The American Neurological Unit and the American Dental Unit

While American personnel staffed hospitals from Villa Paz to the front lines, two other groups of AMBASD volunteers were working as semi-independent units. The American Neurological Unit, headed by Dr. Abraham Ettelson,

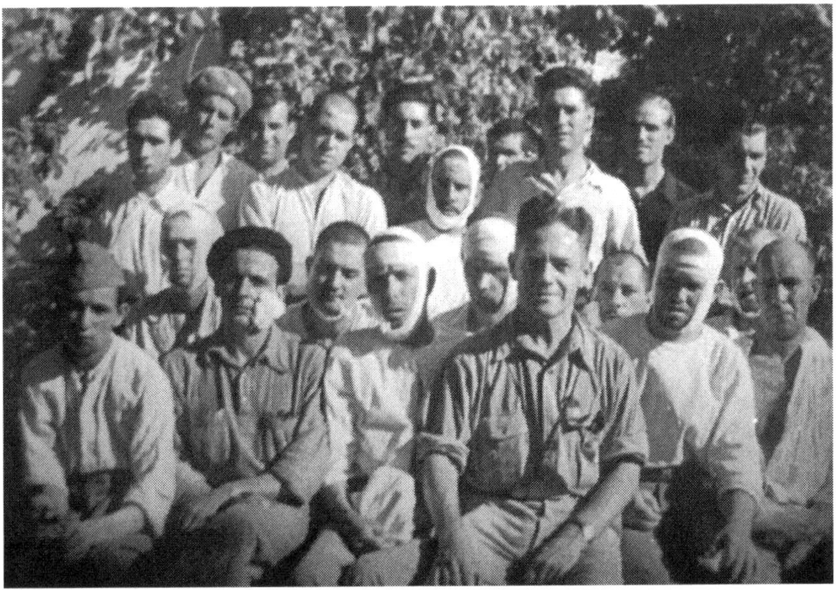

Figure 14. Posner (front, third from right) with patients at Villa Paz (Martin Photograph Collection, Tamiment Library, New York University).

arrived in Spain in the spring of 1937. The group began work at the base hospital and convalescent center of Benicasim until they moved to Godela, on the outskirts of Valencia, in mid-August.[75] In January of 1938, the group moved into the Facultad de Medicina's one-thousand–bed hospital in Valencia, where they had two operating rooms and two large wards.[76] Supported by nearly a dozen Spanish personnel, the group focused on the treatment of head wounds and injuries affecting the vertebral column and peripheral nervous system.

Meanwhile, dentists Donowa, Posner, Stadt, and Klein led the American Dental Unit, treating jaw and facial wounds and also offering routine dental care for soldiers during breaks in fighting.[77] Arriving in the spring of 1937, Posner established himself at Villa Paz, where he treated maxillofacial wounds and extended offerings of dental care to the local population.[78]

Klein and Donowa worked independently in mobile ambulances along the front lines. Despite being closer to the battle, Klein emphasized the routine in later describing that his "job was to spot and prevent teeth that would give trouble in the next year or two."[79] Klein chronicles the removal of five thousand teeth during his stint in Spain. Klein later moved to the American hospital at Vic, north of Barcelona. Klein recalled the difficulty of his job there, particularly given that much of the group's equipment was lost during the hurried evacuation of Villa Paz.

Evacuation: North to Catalonia

As Franco pushed back Republican armed forces, their medical services were forced to evacuate alongside them. Staff had only a few days to organize the evacuation of entire hospitals, including patients, staff, and equipment. Dr. Frances Vanzant remembered receiving the order to evacuate Murcia around 6:00 p.m. on 8 April 1938, with the first patients boarding an evacuation train by 11:00 p.m. that night.[80] The American Dr. Sidney Vogel had been put in charge of the first train while the British doctor, Tudor Hart, was assigned the last. With the patients and staff of more than three different hospitals arriving throughout the night, the station became a scene of confusion as "patients and personnel drifted about . . . without knowing where to go or what to do."[81] The train did not get under way until 6:00 a.m. the next morning, finally arriving in Barcelona around 2:00 a.m. the following Tuesday. Hospitals in Barcelona accommodated many of the new arrivals, while new hospitals were established throughout Catalonia to house and care for the rest. Of these, American volunteers helped organize and staff hospitals at Tortosa, Vallivana, Mataró, and Vic.[82]

About forty kilometers north of Barcelona, the hospital at Vic occupied an eighteenth-century monastery, famous for its paintings and unfortunately, later, a recurrent problem of typhoid. Dr. Barney Malbin was given the task of organizing the hospital's response to an outbreak in April 1938, in which AMBASD volunteer Dr. Leonard Larsen became a patient himself. Aided by the "heroic work" of staff directed by nurses Ruth Davidow and Selma Chadwick, within four days the group had set up "a perfectly organized typhoid ward with complete isolation technique, its own kitchen and utensils, accurate charting and progress notes for all patients and excellent laboratory investigation."[83] Accounts of the resulting mortality rate vary. While Eloesser, in charge of the hospital at Vic, claimed there were no deaths, Larsen guessed there were about a dozen, and dentist Jack Klein reported ten.[84] Still, the outbreak had reportedly been limited to 147 cases (proved by laboratory culture) out of a patient and staff population of nearly 2,000. The outbreak proved interesting from a medical standpoint given that 90 percent of the hospital's population had been immunized against typhoid, and of those with proven infection, 67 percent had received a full vaccine series. [85] Lab technician Dorothy Fontaine also observed the curious incidence of typhoid among "internationals" despite widespread inoculation. Fontaine speculated whether there might be differences in the causative organisms that caused American vaccines to be less effective.[86]

The Demands of Work and Volunteer Health

In volunteers' daily life, more than typhoid put their own health at risk. The intensity of work was highly variable, dependent on shifting battle lines and changes in fighting. Reports of sleepless nights and days on end of feverish work appear throughout volunteer accounts, whether driving ambulances, working in the operating room, or carrying out laboratory duties. Nurse Lini De Vries recalled falling ill one by one in the intensity of their first days at Romeral. "I can remember going off duty with a temperature of 104," De Vries wrote, "And then I remembered no more for two days, except delirium. Delirium with bombs, fascists, anti-fascists, languages, a nightmare."[87]

While De Vries was not the only AMBASD volunteer to spend time in Spain as both patient and staff, few became seriously ill. Early in 1938, Dr. Weisfield had "an upset in his intestinal tract while at the front" and spent a few days at the hospital in Benicasim.[88] Diarrhea and gastrointestinal distress were common for both staff and soldiers, as were dysentery and lice. Nurse Leonora Temple was hospitalized for a number of days with a seriously infected arm.[89] Nurse Esther Silverstein left Spain in 1938 after contracting malaria, undulant fever, and dysentery simultaneously.[90] Dr. Albert Byrne reportedly caught pneumonia after "operating for 6 days and 6 nights without hardly a rest between cases."[91] Jaundice was another frequent complaint, and many also reported returning to the U.S. having lost significant amounts of weight. Dr. Mark Strauss also spent time as a patient, described by Neugass as lying "upstairs on one of the few mattresses; silent, fever-dilated eyes staring upwards, refusing to be evacuated . . . with his lungs . . . gone back on him" and "blue eyes and cheeks bright with fever."[92]

Outside of illness, remarkably few American personnel were wounded. Of the few exceptions, several came during the bombing of a mobile surgical unit at Urrea de Gaen along the Aragon front. Decades later, nurse Anne Taft still remembered the events of that day clearly as she described looking up to see nurse Helen Freeman slumped up against one of the tent poles, her head bleeding profusely.[93] While Freeman's forehead suffered a relatively minor surface wound, her arm was seriously fractured. Although she underwent

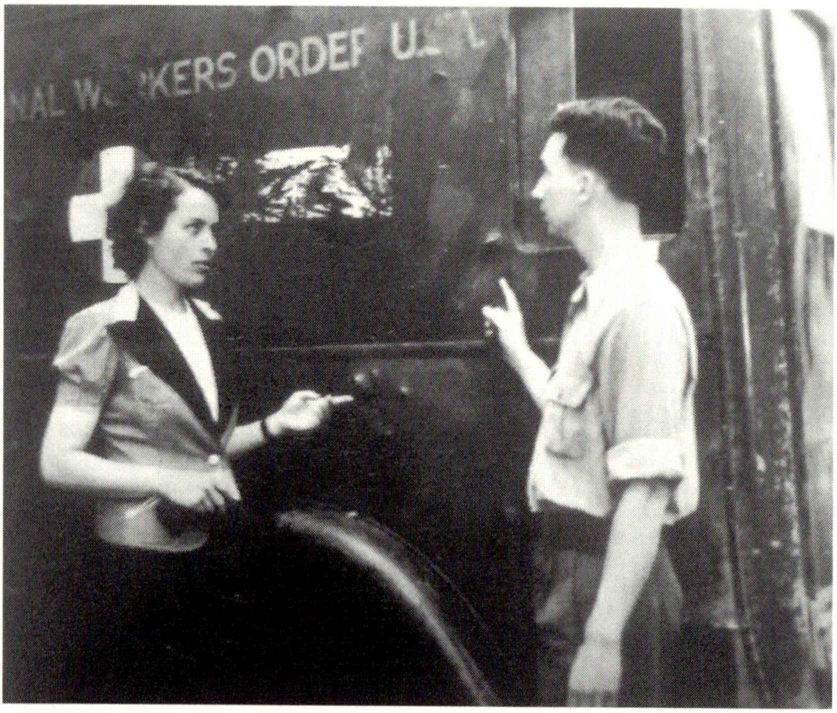

Figure 15. Mildred Rackley (left) and ambulance driver Carl Rahman point out bullet holes in an AMBASD ambulance (Martin Photograph Collection, Tamiment Library, New York University).

several operations to repair the bone and nerve damage, the arm never fully healed.[94] In that same bombing, Cresencia, a Spanish nurse working with the unit, was slightly wounded, and ambulance driver Jack Quiñones broke his leg. Meanwhile, during the bombing of Tarancón in December 1937, nurse Sonia Merims had three ribs fractured from a flying rock while tending to wounded in the street.[95] Ambulance drivers were at even higher personal risk in their routine proximity to the battlefield.

Council Carter, the group's only African American driver, was given a leave of absence to recover from injuries he received.[96] Randall Smith was injured twice, describing one instance of "only flesh wounds" in a letter home.[97] Those same "flesh wounds," however, kept Smith hospitalized for nearly two months.

Down Time

Idle time came in alternation with periods of intense work. During such "periods of idleness," staff cleaned and organized equipment and facilities.[98] "Fiestas" became opportunities for staff and patients to enjoy themselves and were often remembered fondly as examples of the sense of international community and comradery that developed in Spain.[99] American patient Jack Shafran recalled New Year's Eve with great enthusiasm: "We finished off the old year with a bang—we had the first snowfall of the year at the hospital—so—we had a big snowball fight—what fun—(I sprained an ankle so—I am in bed today)—at night we had a small blow out. Just the hospital—it was practically stag—singing songs in about 6 different languages . . . New Year's couldn't be New Years without liquor—you guessed it honey—plenty flowed."[100] Idleness posed an even more constant challenge for patients who were bedridden or hospitalized for long periods of time. One wounded American volunteer, Carl Geiser, wrote home from a Spanish hospital about "a fly-catching session" he and other ward neighbors had to stave off boredom—though unfortunately "even that became dull."[101] Once he had achieved some mobility, Geiser explored the hospital library, where he found a Spanish book of algebra, which he used to "entertain" himself by "extracting cube roots and binomials and dealing with imaginary figures."[102] Another morning, Geiser helped roll bandages for the hospital. At Villa Paz, for a time, there was "almost one staff member for every patient, not because we are overstaffed, but because of the policy of giving easy work to the light wounded."[103] All such pursuits, perhaps with the exception of fly-catching, were common activities for the convalescing patient.

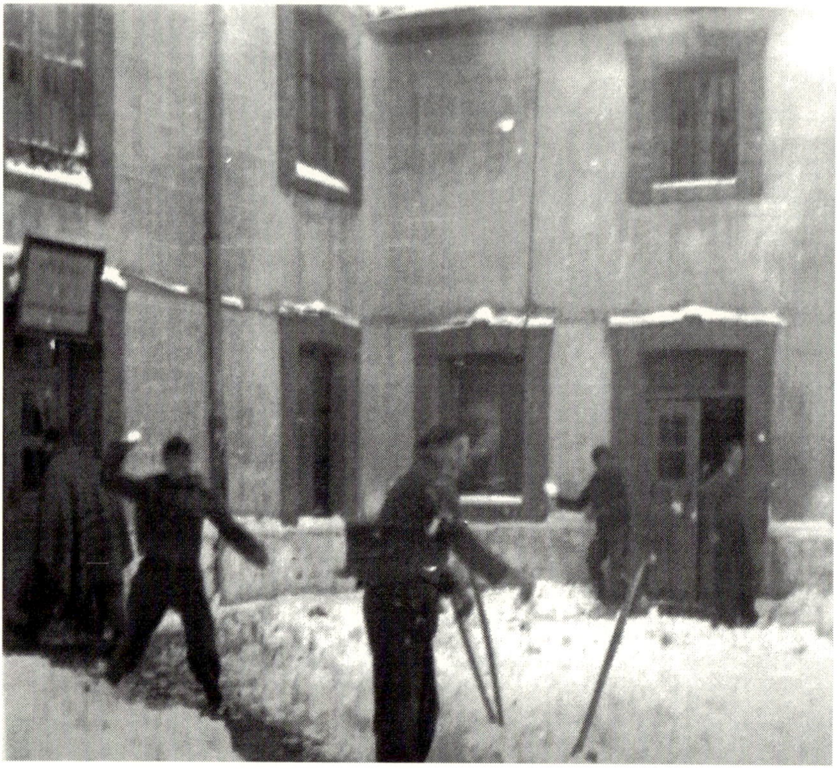

Figure 16. Patients in a snowball fight at Villa Paz (Martin Photograph Collection, Tamiment Library, New York University).

Established convalescent centers, such as Benicasim, tried hard to combat the enforced idleness of the recovering patient. Volunteers formed recreational and educational committees, dedicated to providing opportunities for activities ranging from political discussions to friendly sports matches. At Benicasim, a typical week's events included Spanish classes, news reports, an evening cinema or concert, weekly dances, and hikes in the country.[104] When Geiser was eventually transferred to Benicasim, he was thrilled with the "myriad and one activities" for the convalescent. "Library, writing room, canteen, wall newspapers and in sports, soccer, handball, volleyball, horse shoes, hiking, swimming, tennis and almost anything you can think of," Geiser wrote home.[105] It seemed to matter little to Geiser that most of the sporting opportunities he praises so highly were still off limits to him, due to the injury that had landed him in the hospital in the first place.

Those same periods of idleness, however, could also lead to difficulties among the staff. Recalling getting past the initial rush of wounded at Romeral, De Vries noticed that the group "began being conscious of the food we were eating, chick peas and artichoke hearts, flavored with tough burro meat" and "began griping about things."[106] Rackley similarly described Romeral as becoming a "hotbed of unrest and rumors" as the patient numbers dwindled.[107] News of ongoing inter-staff conflicts even seemed to be reaching New York. When August Towsen left for Spain as an ambulance driver with the fifth unit, he was given the special instructions of sending AMBASD executive secretary Crookston—also Towsen's neighbor in New York—a report of what was going on. Crookston was reportedly concerned about news from AMBASD personnel in Spain "which gave the impression that they were doing nothing but fight among themselves.[108] Towsen later admitted that, "most of the people were acting very immature." While the AMBASD's medical units in Spain were often publicized as images of harmonious industry, the reality seems to have been much more variable.

While the volunteer units of the Spanish Civil War may have established a new precedent in racial integration, tensions remained. Although it's not clear what, if any, role it had in her departure, Martin apparently had a falling out with African American nurse Salaria Kee, who had charged Martin with racial discrimination. According to Martin, the disagreement had arisen after she had been encouraged by Dr. Busch to persuade Kee to postpone her impending marriage with Irish International Brigader Pat O'Reilly.[109] Despite the AMBASD's use of Kee as a public image of the progressive and open-minded nature of their endeavor—the first racially integrated military medical division in U.S. history—Kee described difficulties. Crossing the Atlantic to Spain, the doctor in charge of her group had apparently refused to sit at the same table as her. Kee reported that the ship's captain instead invited her to dine at his table, which she continued to do for the rest of the voyage.[110]

In several other cases, personal disagreements seemed to directly affect the movement of AMBASD personnel. A reportedly "unfair dislike" of Mildred Rackley for her "formal manners" and general "jealousy of her close friendship with Barsky" seems to have been a contributing factor in her decision to leave Villa Paz to help the British set up a hospital at Huete.[111] Personal disagreements contributed to the movement of other personnel too, as lab technician Dorothy Fontaine accounted for her move to Belalcazar from Villa Paz as a result of her inability to get along with colleague Rose Freed.[112] Dentist John Posner appears in accounts as another controversial figure at Villa Paz.

Having reportedly instigated a movement to establish separate dining tables for staff and patients, a series of questionnaires were circulated among AMBASD personnel to gauge interest and support. Nearly all voiced strong opposition to the idea, with one respondent suggesting simply that the best way to improve conditions at the hospital would be to "squash Dr. Posner."[113] Many protested that the proposal ran counter to the principles of equality and cooperation that were fundamental to many volunteer beliefs.

There has been little found written from Posner's point of view, although reports suggest that he ultimately left Spain after six months feeling "disgusted" with the Communist influence in the medical services.[114] Posner was, however, attributed with the authorship on one of the more creatively satirical pieces to emerge from AMBASD volunteers. Writing on the imagined species of the "Americana infermera":

> Was first seen in Spain in the early part of February, 1937. Noted for its clear bell like trill or call, especially among the females of 'Americasbest' repeated at frequent intervals. It is most gregarious, but strongly resents the intrusion of any foreign species into its lair, or nest. Noted for 'its' voracious habits of frequently indulging in nocturnal feasts, to which a few chosen males are sometimes invited. Is very addicted to certain drinks or beverages, notably the juice of a plant called grape, or in its more potent form, "champagne." Frequently suffers from real pain afterwards. Plumage. Usually blue or white, with a ruff around the neck of contrasting color. Will not breed well in captivity. Is of a delicate constitution, which makes it almost impossible for it to acclimatize itself in a foreign climate.[115]

Posner was not the only one to note the abundance of wine in Spain—and volunteers' general willingness to take advantage of it. As Martin wrote simply of her own progress on recording the history of AMBASD volunteers in Spain, "if I were to put down" every episode in which "a staff member was drunk I would need to write in ten volumes."[116] Not all interpreted the nurse's romantic tendencies with such vitriol. As noted by Neugass, with the "strings of admirers" the nurses attracted, "many of the men are put to sleep at night by a sedative dreaminess of unrequited love, thus saving us much luminal."[117]

Meanwhile, nurse Toby Jensky appears to have been one of the inspiring figures for Posner's piece of creative writing. Alluding to a similar episode in letters home during the summer of 1937:

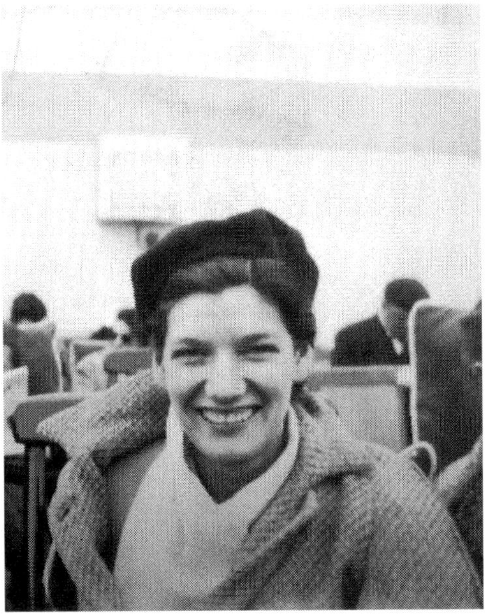

Figure 17. Toby Jensky on the S.S. Normandie on her way to Spain (Jensky Photograph Collection, Tamiment Library, New York University).

> As for me—I'm doing well and am contented—for a while all the girls were very much disgruntled—it seems that a couple of sex starved old fogies decided we were immoral and put down some silly rules for us—which we resented—I didn't come to Spain to be made a lady of—Before this we and anybody else we invited used to get together in the nurses quarters usually my room and eat and gab—one of the rules is—no men allowed in our rooms—what they expected us to do with 3+ girls in each room—I'm hanged. Anyway the rules still stand—but what the hell—so we have more to eat ourselves.[118]

Despite such rules, Jensky described enjoying a number of romantic intrigues during her time in Spain, mostly with patients among the International Brigades. First there was the Czech she met in Barcelona, then the English sculptor—"about 6 ft 2—blond—very mod," and later the American with whom she had "more of a cat and mouse affair."[119] The English sculptor was her "big romance" and the two were nearly married in Spain. After the war was over, Jensky visited him in England, where they married in spite of skeptical letters home.

Jensky was not the only one to find matrimony in Spain. Salaria Kee married Irish International Brigader Pat O'Reilly. Irene Goldin married an Austrian brigader.[120] Ave Bruzzichesi married Lincoln Brigader A. Wolfman.[121] Nurse Thelma Erickson and Dr. Albert Byrne were married in Valencia on

22 February 1938.[122] Dr. Philip Goland reportedly married a Spanish student nurse in Valencia.[123] Becky Schulman also supposedly married a Spaniard during her time abroad. Even when romances didn't result in marriage, they could be a source of tension among the staff as a whole, with rumors running rampant.[124] As nurse Mary Platkin lamented at Benicasim, "Everybody in this little dizzy place knows who we are going out with and where."[125]

Interpersonal complications and the problems that they may have caused were not limited to the Americans in Spain. As Celia Greenspan wrote from another international hospital, "Unfortunately we have too many surgeons here now and they act like prima donnas," causing "an undercurrent of ill feeling and dissension." But thankfully, Greenspan continued, "My German is so bad that no one bothers to tell me all the lurid details of what this one said to whom and the outcome of petty triumphs and defeats."[126] Dr. A. L. Cochrane, of the British unit, admitted that in addition to political conflicts, "the big social differences between members of the unit," the "fair amount of sleeping about with all the consequent jealousies," and the lack of sufficient work all led to personnel difficulties at the British hospital in Grañen.[127]

Sometimes personal conflicts and rivalries had more serious consequences. The circumstances surrounding the arrest of Dr. Albert Byrne by Republican authorities in the spring of 1938 are still somewhat shrouded in mystery, but discord within the ranks of AMBASD personnel may have been

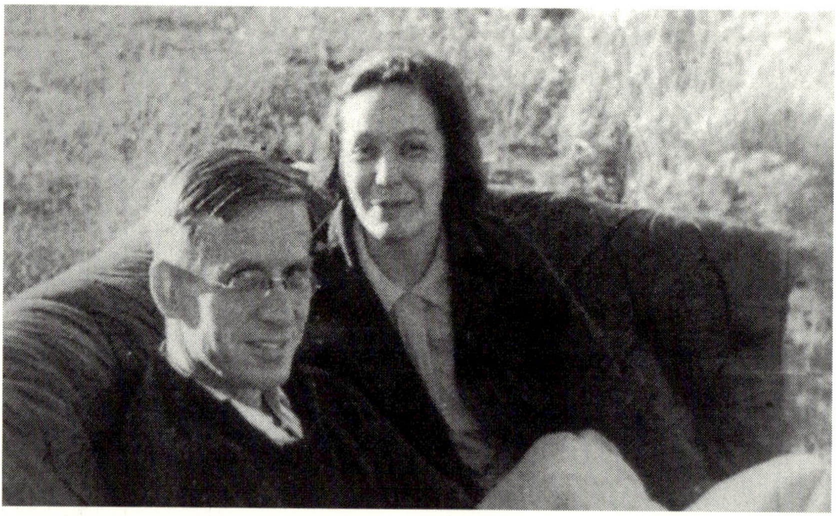

Figure 18. Dr. Albert Byrne and nurse Thelma Erickson in Spain (Martin Photograph Collection, Tamiment Library, New York University).

a contributing factor. Byrne's arrest followed his return to Valencia from falling ill at the front in February, where he joined fiancée and nurse Thelma Erickson working in the neurological unit. The couple married soon after and reportedly began trying to secure leave to return home. Some colleagues reported that under Thelma's influence Byrne began denouncing the Republic, while others argue that it was another American doctor within the unit who wrongly reported him to authorities for questionable loyalties. A contemporary report noted simply that, "according to authorities . . . Dr. Byrne was arrested because of his unwillingness to recognize that doctors, like soldiers, must consider themselves militarized."[128] Whatever the reasons behind it, Byrne was eventually released.

The political climate in Valencia seems to have been particularly unfavorable for AMBASD volunteers, as nurses Leonora Temple and Cleo Duncan were also arrested there and imprisoned for a short period of time. The American consul in Valencia, Woodruff Wallner, was able to secure their release after only a few days. Both were preparing to leave Spain to return home and, as Wallner reported, "foreigners desiring to leave Spain . . . inevitably arouse the suspicion of the authorities."[129] Meanwhile, Republican authorities apparently arrested African American nurse Salaria Kee, suspecting she was a Nationalist "moor" in disguise.[130] Although Kee was released promptly, the episode is still an interesting indication of Spanish racial perspectives and prejudices at the time.

The details surrounding the death of pharmacist Harry Wilkes are even murkier. Wilkes initially traveled to Spain with the first AMBASD unit and, after taking a personal leave in the fall of 1937, returned in January 1938. When he did not return to the U.S. again as expected the following summer, his family began making inquiries. Reporting back to AMBASD headquarters in July 1938, Dr. Sidney Vogel wrote, "Wilkes died a heroic death on the front while fulfilling his duties in defense of liberty and the Republic of Spain."[131] Only much later was this story discounted in light of new records suggesting that Republican authorities in fact executed Wilkes for his alleged participation in black market schemes involving drugs, currency, and fine art.[132]

Perceptions of Americans in Spain

The reputation of American nurses as poor at acclimatizing to their foreign situation lampooned in the "Americana infermera" resonates with other accounts. In her research after the war, Martin noted that some European

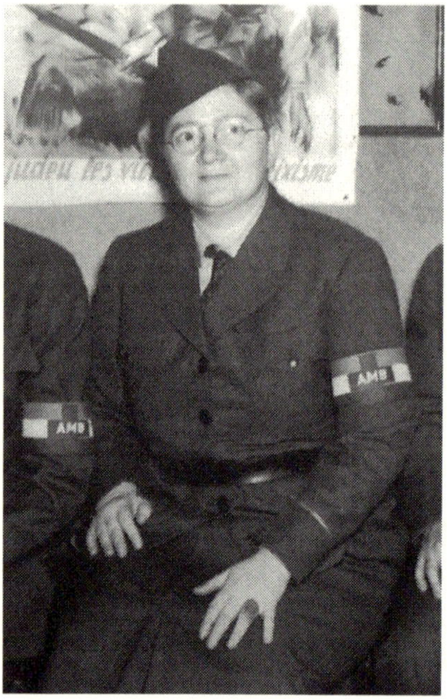

Figure 19. Dr. Frances Vanzant, in AMBASD uniform (Martin Photograph Collection, Tamiment Library, New York University).

colleagues still resented the "separatism" of U.S. doctors and nurses. While acknowledging a valid base for their attitude, Martin also noted, "They just don't realize how knowing only English and being slow to pick up other languages debarred us gals from intimacy."[133] Martin described Villa Paz, in particular, as encouraging U.S. isolationism among the volunteers. The atmosphere there was "contaminated" by a "fear of leaving the womb which affected most of the female personnel and most of the doctors," an unfortunate circumstance even if "the base of the fear was understandable . . . with the poor facility most U.S. people have for dominating another language and having assumed that they were to be in American hospitals and groups."[134]

Despite their reputation of being linguistically ill-equipped, a number of U.S. volunteers worked outside of predominantly American teams. After Eloesser returned to the U.S., Ave Bruzzichesi became head operating room nurse for a Spanish surgeon.[135] Esther Silverstein stepped into a similar role for famous Catalan surgeon, Moises Broggi, after having worked with the British at Huete, along with Irene Goldin.[136] Shortly after her arrival in Spain, Dr. Frances Vanzant was placed in charge of a hospital in Murcia.

Vanzant was the only American in her hospital and later recalled the challenges of taking over without knowing any Spanish. When she arrived she had only three English-speaking patients and fewer than a dozen of her staff spoke any English.[137] Despite the challenges, Vanzant spoke highly of her experience. Her arrival itself was "heralded and well received," as the chief doctor introduced her the next day to patients and staff as "a distinguished doctor from the U.S., very famous." For Vanzant, "the build-up" was "very helpful . . . straddled with the difficulty of knowing no language except English."[138] Those who did speak languages other than English—such as Hartmann, De Vries, and Brisker—found themselves able to make valuable contributions working among non-English speaking nationalities.

AMBASD volunteers report developing relationships with a number of local communities. Dr. Julius Hene wrote home about the popularity of the Americans in one town: "We have developed an enormous practice with the townspeople and the peasants. They stream in all through siesta to have scratches dressed. Every kid in town comes in regularly every day to have his knees bandaged with the latest Johnson & Johnson lenkoplast contraptions and politically we can't refuse them."[139] For Hene, American medicine served as a bridge—socially and politically—to connecting with the Spanish people. Other Spaniards, as well, echo the novelty of the American presence described by Hene in their own memories.[140] Some towns went out of their way to assist the American effort. In Romeral, when Rackley complained about the terrible condition of the roads connecting the front to Romeral for the transportation of the wounded, the *alcaldes* of Romeral and a neighboring village gathered groups of locals to repair them.[141] De Vries said later that villagers were practically fighting one another for the opportunity to help the Americans, be it in the kitchen, as nurses' aides, or assistants to the drivers and mechanics.[142] Meanwhile, in Belalcazar, nurse Anne Shuldiner remembered a "mixed reception from the community," with "cordiality and support from the *alcalde* and councillors and shopkeepers," but scant acknowledgement from the "people from the beautiful homes . . . when we walked or rode by and greeted them."[143]

In his description of Villa Paz, Neugass also highlights some of the complexities in the reception of American aid by local people. While proudly proclaiming what "American money, American technical skill, American hands and sweat have helped the Spanish establish and organize," Neugass went on to mention some friction with the local physician: "Peasants come to us from all Cuenca province with the ills which have afflicted them for centuries, expecting miracles. The Saelices doctor . . . complains that we are taking away his trade. He is so unfamiliar with modern medicine that it would be unwise for us to take him in with us or to set him up in a village clinic."[144] The account given by Neugass sharply contrasts the limitations of Spanish medicine and resources with the wealth of material and knowledge of the American volunteer unit. In comparison to other accounts of the glowing local reception, one must wonder what the Saelices doctor Neugass describes might have said about the AMBASD presence. Other accounts suggest strong professional ties were developed between local Spaniards and the visiting AMBASD volunteers, with Americans and Spaniards working alongside one another in a number of hospitals and mobile units. Many American nurses involved in training Spanish *chicas* in modern nursing developed particularly close friendships with their new colleagues.[145] Neugass suggests this investment in training was also intentional. Writing from Alcorisa in January, he said, "We plan to leave our skill in Spain, not only our bodies. A Spanish expert is now being trained to take over the management of the garage" and "Spanish are put into responsible positions . . . as fast as they can be secured."[146]

From Republicans to Refugees

Over the winter of 1938–1939, there appeared a flash of broader concern for the victims of the Spanish conflict, both from the U.S. government and the ARC. In November 1938, the *Erica Reed* set sail for Spain, laden with $250,000 worth of food and relief supplies from multiple sources—including the ARC, American Friends Service Committee (AFSC), and Federal Surplus Commodities Corporation.[147] That winter, President Roosevelt appointed a committee directed to help the ARC and AFSC provide "impartial" civilian relief in Spain. The committee hoped to gather $500,000 to be applied to the cost of shipments of wheat to Spain, but only raised $50,000. Roosevelt reportedly considered taking even more proactive measures, but was advised against doing so by congressional and State Department advisors.[148] In spite of some efforts to encourage undercover military operations on Spanish soil, there seemed to be little to be done in the absence of any dramatic change in policy.[149] Although Roosevelt told pressure groups that American policy in Spain "had been a grave mistake," Nationalist victory was nearly secured.[150]

Despite the brief rise in activity in the months before, once Barcelona had fallen to Nationalist forces in January 1939, the national network of humanitarian relief assembled by the North American Committee had crumbled.[151] As the Nationalists closed in on the last pocket of Republican territory, the movement of refugees to France intensified. Between the last week of January and first week of February more than 450,000 refugees crossed the border into France.[152] Nurse Ave Bruzzichesi later described the evacuation as "the most impressive" and "most heartbreaking episode of the entire war."[153] The scene was exacerbated by the French government's lack of preparation for the huge influx of refugees. Once across the border, refugees were gathered into camps with reportedly terrible conditions. By the time Bruzzichesi left, "a typhoid epidemic had started at St. Cyprian, a diphtheria epidemic at Camp Arles . . . and many died from lack of food and the cold."[154] After entering France, Bruzzichesi joined a British group offering medical care to refugees in the camps.[155]

On 1 April 1939, Francisco Franco declared victory following the surrender of the last Republican forces. London and Paris officially recognized the Nationalist government on 27 February 1939 and Washington followed suit on 3 April 1939.[156] A handful of AMBASD volunteers—such as Bruzzichesi—remained as workers in these camps, while others sought to rejuvenate relief efforts in the U.S. by reorienting the discourse toward the plight of the refugees. But for the majority of AMBASD volunteers, however, the end of the war meant a return to the United States.

Conclusions

The presence of the AMBASD's volunteers in Spain afforded a small group of Americans a unique perspective of the Spanish Civil War. As much political debate as their work may have inspired over the significance of the AMBASD for U.S. foreign relations, their experiences were by and large much more immediate to the concerns of their professions and the realities of life in a war zone. The highly personal experiences of volunteers transformed the significance of their time abroad. For some it inspired greater political activism, while encouraging others to seek out other experiences in medical volunteerism. While there was the impetus for organizing ABMAC's efforts on a similar foundation of medical volunteers to China, such work never took off in the same way. While many factors contributed to this difference in organizational practices between the AMBASD and the ABMAC, the chronological backdrop of World War II played a major role. With huge amounts of manpower and resources being devoted directly to the American war effort, the availability of would-be volunteers changed significantly. The more global war also fundamentally changed the prospects for the type of medical activism initially pursued by the AMBASD and the ABMAC, which relied on private and independently organized action.

CHAPTER FIVE

Avenues of Aid for Americans in China

While the volunteer movement mounted by the AMBASD came to define its practical identity, the medical relief orchestrated by private groups in aid of China lacked a parallel dimension. Although Robert Lim of the CRC had encouraged the ABMAC to send medical volunteers, ABMAC-sponsored medical personnel remained limited to a handful of individuals. The ABMAC found greater success in responding to Lim's request to help fund the return journeys of a couple of dozen Chinese physicians, nurses, and medical personnel studying in the United States. Similarly, although the CAC helped coordinate the travel of a few medical volunteers to serve alongside Chinese Communist forces, numbers were limited.

Private U.S. aid efforts provided an avenue for some Americans to become witnesses to the escalating conflict in East Asia, but organizations such as the ABMAC and CAC did not hold as unique a position as the AMBASD in offering a route for private citizens to travel into distant conflict zones. In China, many of the Americans who became involved in private aid efforts were already there. And those who were sent through the private aid channels discussed in this study were more often organizational representatives, helping orchestrate the logistics of aid, rather than medical professionals treated the wounded or sick. For others, traditional national military channels offered a more direct route to medical service in conflict zones.

ABMAC Volunteers

Throughout the extensive correspondence that developed between the CRC and the ABMAC, the need for medical personnel became a recurring theme. As noted by Lim in a letter to Co Tui in 1941, "There is certainly an important need for personnel in China and ABMAC will be doing great service if aid can be given to alleviate the shortage of personnel."[1] By that same year, ABMAC leadership declared that the organization was entering its "fourth stage" of relief work.[2] Having addressed shortages of emergency supplies, medical equipment, and transportation supplies in its first three stages, the problem of personnel became its next priority.

By January 1942, the ABMAC's Board of Directors had begun discussing plans to send a cadre of volunteers. Lim had particularly emphasized the need for general surgeons (especially in orthopedics), nursing supervisors, and experts in public health. But although money had been allocated to staff volunteer units, "wartime conditions" were blamed for "making volunteers hard to come by."[3] The ABMAC's selectivity did not help. In that same meeting, a number of names were reported as being under consideration, but few of these met the medical committee's basic linguistic and professional requirements.[4] The application for medical, technical, or dental service in China with ABMAC required applicants to report basic biographical and professional training, in addition to any ROTC or military experience. Candidates were required to submit two references and a medical report. The application form made explicit that volunteers would be accepted for a two-year commitment, either as a medical officer or technician under the National Red Cross Society of China or National Health Administration of China.[5] Only those with an M.D. would be considered, automatically disqualifying a group of sixteen to eighteen osteopathic doctors who volunteered in the spring of 1942.[6]

In the months (and years) that followed, the number of those rejected for service in China exceeded the number of those accepted. Contacts in China expressed concern over the abilities of potential American volunteers to withstand local conditions. Dr. Leo Eloesser, who had served with the AMBASD in Spain, had volunteered to assemble a small unit including himself, an intern, and two nurses.[7] However, following reports from the Chinese ambassador suggesting that the kinds of equipment needed by Eloesser would not likely be available and that conditions in China might exceed Eloesser's constitution, the offer was turned down by the ABMAC Medical Committee.[8] In 1945, just as World War II came to an end, Eloesser traveled to China under United Nations auspices to teach surgery, becoming involved in the training of China's "barefoot doctors."[9]

Despite the string of rejections, a few American volunteers did travel to China through ABMAC channels. Dr. Adele Cohn, a specialist in tuberculosis, arrived in China in 1941. Dentist R. Gordon Agnew, who would later write a report on dental education in China for the Chinese Ministry of Health, personally escorted thirty cases of surgical and dental instruments, a dental x-ray machine, twenty-two microfilm readers, and two microscopes to China via India.[10] Dr. John Scudder, a specialist in blood transfusion and surgery at Columbia University's College of Physicians and Surgeons, also traveled to China with an ABMAC-organized blood bank. Two Chinese physicians studying under Scudder in New York also traveled with him—Dr. Helena Wong, and Dr. Chien-Lung Yi.[11]

Prior to his involvement with the ABMAC, Scudder developed a similar blood transfusion program in Great Britain. In late 1939, Scudder and Charles R. Drew, a former graduate student in his research lab, began setting up Blood for Britain.[12] At that time, the use of plasma (the liquid component of blood holding blood cells in suspension) as a substitute for whole blood in transfusions was still in its early days. However, Scudder and Drew had proven that plasma could be refrigerated and stored for up to two months, in addition to beginning work with dried plasma formulations. The Blood Transfusion Betterment Association of New York recruited them to design a program that would send American plasma and transfusion techniques to Britain through the American Red Cross. Drew (an African American) later became the medical director for the program, a pioneering role considering that the first pilot project had excluded black donors at the insistence of the armed forces, and even in its later stages kept donations made by whites and blacks segregated.[13] (Interestingly, imagery used in ABMAC promotional

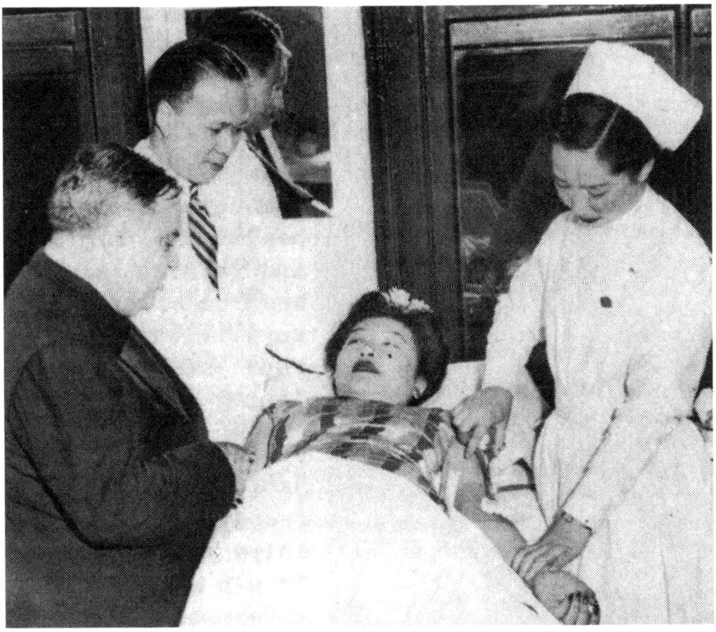

Figure 20. Mayor La Guardia (of New York City) attends an opening of a blood bank for China (USC Records, Mudd Manuscript Library, Princeton University).

material of an ABMAC blood bank in the U.S. appears segregated, although some records of volunteer numbers contradict the image, with as many white donors as other ethnic backgrounds.)

Although ABMAC plans for the blood bank began in the early 1940s, it took several years for the unit to get underway. Nevertheless, on 12 July 1944, the blood bank began operations in Kunming.[14] A few days before the ABMAC team departed, each U.S. and Chinese member was given a commission in the Chinese army.[15] General Ma, the representative of China's Ministry of War, was the first donor, and in the week following its opening, the blood bank registered more than twenty thousand soldiers, students, and college professors.[16] Such numbers suggest that Western medical traditions had gained enough of a foothold in China by this point to minimize controversy over the practice within traditional Chinese medicine. Americans present in China spoke highly of the blood bank's impact. As General Joseph Stilwell wrote to Dr. Van Slyke in 1944, "The Chinese Bloodbank . . . has been extending a grand service to the brave and tenacious Chinese soldiers in the Yoke Forces," and "many soldiers have been saved by the fine work of your organization." For Stilwell, the power of the blood bank went beyond its medical work. "Everything possible," Stilwell continued, "will be done to keep this humanitarian project a powerful weapon which will long be remembered."[17]

Scudder himself traveled to China in 1945 with two nurses returning to China from studies in the U.S., Mrs. Elsie Chung Lyon and Miss Margaret Tchou, and 1,200 pounds of equipment. Upon arrival, Scudder was surprised at the great backlogs of medical supplies stuck in Kunming. Although the ARC had helped to move many of these supplies, microfilms, books, and other ABMAC donations remained unused.[18] As a physician and volunteer in a small American relief organization, Scudder achieved remarkable access to important people and places during his visit. In May, Scudder wrote to UCR president Charles Edison:

> I have just returned from China where I have been working with the Chinese Blood Bank, having been requested to go to China by the former Chinese Surgeon-General Hsu Hsilin. While working there, I went with a convoy down into the valleys. I saw the Army hospitals . . . I visited what was called a 200 bed hospital which had neither a nurse nor a doctor to take care of the wounded . . . I also went to Chungking where I had an interview with the Generalissimo. In that interview, the Generalissimo expressed his appreciation

> of ABMAC's program. He told me of the needs of his soldiers for better medical care; of his hope that the ABMAC would continue to help in improving and strengthening the Army hospitals and urged that ABMAC increase its aid toward the medical care of his soldiers.[19]

At this point, the ABMAC reportedly had plans underway to send $50,000 in donations to China through the U.S. Army. (Although Van Slyke later contested this.) The U.S. Army could transfer money at a more favorable exchange rate (by a difference of about 33 percent), which made many aid agencies eager to find a way to use this channel to transmit funds. However, as UCR president Edison noted, the ABMAC's plans were questionable because "if either the Chinese or American government discovered that we were using the U.S. Army as a channel for transmitting our relief funds to China we would at once get into serious trouble."[20] Edison clearly drew a distinction between UCR's intention of transferring "non-governmental funds given for relief purposes" rather than "governmental funds used in carrying on direct war effort."[21] In the end, it appears that the ABMAC found other channels for transferring the money that it raised.

Meanwhile, as China continued facing manpower shortages, the ABMAC continued to investigate ways of addressing this need. Forkner, speaking to the steering committee of UCR as early as 1942, argued that priority should be to get Chinese doctors back, to get missionary doctors and nurses back, and to line up reserved U.S. Army or Navy doctors for service. Forkner's prioritization of China even led him to suggest that draft-age American medical personnel might be assigned first for military duty in China rather than the U.S.[22] By UCR's estimation, such a medical mission could become highly important for the war effort, helping protect both the Chinese army and the Chinese populace.

The recruitment of Chinese physicians as volunteers for the Chinese Red Cross Society represented a conscious change in policy. Although initially searching for American personnel, the ABMAC medical committee encountered difficulties finding American volunteers of the abilities and caliber requested by Lim. As outlined by one member of the medical committee, "Originally Dr. Lim had asked us to send him quite a number of American experts. However, as soon as America got into the war it became increasingly difficult to find and send the type of American personnel he wanted."[23]

One network that became extremely important was that of the Rockefeller Foundation, whose presence in China and established educational exchanges had created a ready-made community of highly trained Chinese medical personnel on temporary study-abroad programs. As of April 1942, the Rockefeller Foundation was sponsoring at least twenty-seven Chinese fellows in the U.S., including ten from the PUMC. However, few showed interest in returning to China. In fact, reporting in 1942, only one "[wanted] to return to China immediately or in the near future."[24]

Dr. Marion Yang had been born in 1891 at the American Board Mission. She earned her M.D. in 1917 at the Union Women's Medical College and pursued specialty training in obstetrics and gynecology at the PUMC in the 1920s. Later studying in England and in the U.S. (at Johns Hopkins), Yang split time between the U.S. and China over the following two decades.[25] Returning to China to serve on the faculty of the PUMC, Yang returned to the U.S. for further studies on a Rockefeller Foundation fellowship in the late 1930s or early 1940s. Yet as the war escalated, a strong sense of duty called her back to China. As she described to the ABMAC Medical Committee: "I am still anxious to return as soon as possible, unless I can render some useful service to the war by remaining in this country . . . In peace-time, I will be very happy in settling down and study for a period of years in this country. When in war-time, trained as a physicians and a position held as mine and stay away from duties, feel somewhat guilty. In addition, I might influence a number of Chinese doctors to return, if I return myself."[26] Yang returned to China in the early autumn of 1942, along with Dr. Ping Yang Liu.[27] Both Yang and Liu had been in the U.S. on Rockefeller Foundation-funded activities, and had their return financed by the ABMAC and Rockefeller Foundation.

Although the ABMAC guaranteed their salaries, volunteers were to be paid directly by the Chinese Red Cross Society—with American volunteers to be paid at a higher rate than Chinese volunteers. New medical graduates were to receive $25 per month; established doctors, $75 per month; and Chinese specialists or heads of department, $150 per month.[28] American specialists were to receive potentially different salaries, arranged individually but promised to be higher than rates offered by the mission boards.[29] For some potential Chinese recruits, this difference in standards and pay were significant, and the conditions offered deemed insufficient for their own living conditions and career ambitions. Dr. Margaret Hie Ding Lin, for instance, first contacted Co Tui in November 1941, writing from the University of Illinois (where she was completing her PhD) of her desire to return to China. She noted her desire to return based on the conditions of "*modern* living quarters, a good salary, and transportation paid"—a standard of living "just like the missionaries."[30] The committee's ultimately recommended ending negotiations with her, based on the idea "that Dr. Lin's demands were not in line with the spirit in which doctors should go out to serve on Dr. Lim's staff."[31] One Chinese physician, Dr. Shu Chu Chen, working as a tuberculosis specialist in the U.S., would only return on the condition that he be able to institute his tuberculosis plan for China—a plan that received a low priority amid China's wartime demands. Helena Wong would only return "by aeroplane" if "placed in charge of a clinical lab or medical clinic or allowed to practice or teach parasitology . . . under the Chinese Red Cross."[32]

Despite difficulties recruiting Chinese working or studying in the U.S., a cadre of physicians and medical personnel was eventually gathered. All but one of these ten were Chinese.[33] Meanwhile, the recruitment of American personnel was put on hold in the autumn of 1943. Both Dr. Bachman and Columbia physician and tuberculosis specialist Dr. Adele Cohn reported "present conditions" in China being such as to "make it almost impossible . . . to consider sending American nurses through India to China."[34] Writing to the ABMAC from China in September 1943, Dr. Cohn reported:

> I feel honestly that my work here is useful and after two years apprenticeship in adaptation and understanding Chinese patients it would be a pity to go home. I do hope the board can see their way clear to increase my salary since it is trying to live under these not-too-easy conditions and to have perpetual worries about making the proverbial ends meet. I honestly can tell you I have sold everything I can possibly sell to increase my funds and I do not want to part with necessary things.[35]

Supported by the ABMAC, Dr. Cohn had joined the Chinese Red Cross as a volunteer. Meanwhile, over a year later, a group of six more Chinese physicians and medical scientists studying in the U.S. (including Marion Yang) still had yet to leave.

Another group the ABMAC discussed actively seeking out for volunteers included mission boards with activities in China.[36] Ruth Derr, a registered nurse who traveled to China as a volunteer funded by the ABMAC, spoke Chinese from having been born in China to an American missionary family. Scudder also came from a missionary family who had spent extensive time in India. As discussed in Chapter 1, the ABMAC found a ready community of support in the U.S. amid those with missionary ties to China. Some, like Walter B. Judd, became extremely vocal supporters both of the ABMAC and Nationalist cause, based on their experiences in China. Not all, however, would share the same political orientation from their time abroad, and the CAC and Chinese Red Cross also found a number of supporters among missionary communities in the Northwest.

In China as a missionary and teacher at Central China College, John B. Foster became a vocal supporter of the Chinese Communists and volunteered with the Chinese Red Cross Society. Watching the growing conflict with Japan, Foster's pacifism turned toward activism, and his initial sympathies for the Nationalist government shifted in favor of the Chinese Communists.[37] Between 1937 and 1939, Foster discussed military and political affairs with a number of Chinese leaders. By early 1938, Foster was discussing his hope that "perhaps it is in China that we shall see first the synthesis of Communism and Christianity."[38] Foster became involved in refugee relief in Hankow through the Chinese Red Cross, Northwestern Partisan Relief Committee, and China Defence League. He also traveled with the Eighth Route Army to Shansi, where he served in a Red Cross hospital until personnel were evacuated following Japanese occupation. His "activist" interests, however, got him into trouble with mission and college officials. Choosing to resign from Central China College, Foster returned to the U.S., working for the U.S. Information Service in the late 1940s.[39] He tried to publish parts of his China journal in 1938, but had his work rejected. Publishers argued that too much of his work focused on discussing Communism, without offering enough first hand material about the Chinese people.

Canadian nurse Jean Ewen first traveled to China in 1933 through missionary means, although without Foster's deeply religious motivations. "The Canada we were leaving behind," Ewen later wrote, "was locked in the Depression, and as recently graduated nurses, we were lucky to have a job of any sort, let alone one that promised such great adventure."[40] Moving between mission stations at Changtien, Kiang Kia, and Chu Li Chang, Ewen picked up an impressive command of the Chinese language and set up a number of dispensaries to great acclaim among mission staff. However, she confessed to being far from a missionary herself. "I could not be," Ewen wrote, "for the spirit of self-denial most certainly wasn't part of my make-up. I did things because I wanted to do them, it was that uncomplicated."[41] Joining local celebrations after Chiang Kai-shek agreed to sign the articles of the United Front, Ewen told of her desire to join the Eighth Route Army.[42]

Nevertheless, in June 1937 she and two friends (also nurses) returned to Canada. Ewen was home less than a year before once again en route to China. The descriptions of her motivations resonate strongly with many of those offered by AMBASD volunteers in their choices to travel to Spain—almost more so than the generally more professionally oriented arguments made by the ABMAC's volunteers.

CAC Volunteers

In contrast to the ABMAC, one of the first priorities of the CAC involved arranging for a handful of individuals—including Ewen—to travel to China as medical volunteers. Like ABMAC volunteers, they were to join units of the Chinese Red Cross society, although they were sent only to the Northwest. Not long after reading an article by Agnes Smedley describing the horrors of civilian bombing, Ewen received a mimeographed appeal from Smedley, passed on by her sister Isobel, for medical personnel to serve in China. After a brief internal debate, Ewen reported to the Communist Party Headquarters the following day. Ewen then traveled to New York City, where the CAC administered a psychological screening assessing her motives. In New York, she met Dr. Norman Bethune for the first time, along with other CAC staff, at the home of the American League for Peace and Democracy.[43] The original American contingent of their party, Dr. Fraad, had been replaced by Dr. Parsons—who would end up separating from Bethune and Ewen in China, effectively transforming the American-Canadian unit into simply a Canadian one.[44]

Before traveling to China in 1938, Bethune had served Republican forces in Spain, helping to set up a mobile blood transfusion service based out of Madrid.[45] When the reorganization of the Sanidad Militar was announced in the spring of 1937, Bethune was deeply frustrated by the loss of autonomy of foreign medical units.[46] However, funds for the transfusion service he had established were still needed. Returning to Canada in the summer of 1937, Bethune toured North America, speaking on behalf of the Spanish cause. Reading news of the developing conflict in China, Bethune became inspired by a new cause. With the military situation in Spain having deteriorated, and Bethune feeling his speaking tour had achieved all that it could, he wrote to the Spanish Aid Committee in Toronto that his efforts were needed more directly elsewhere.[47]

Bethune arrived in Hong Kong on 20 January 1938, partly supported by the CAC.[48] After arriving in Yenan, Lebanese-American physician Dr.

George Hatem helped Bethune establish medical services for the front lines. Having traveled to China independently in 1933, Hatem joined the Chinese Communist Party and dedicated the rest of his life to practicing medicine in China.[49] He traveled (secretly) with friend and journalist Ed Snow, whose book *Red Star Over China* became one of the first introductions of Mao Zedong and the Chinese Communists to the English-speaking world. Snow described Hatem as "beneath a superficial cynicism serious about one thing" in wanting to "find his purpose as a doctor."[50] Like himself, Snow concluded, Hatem had found that purpose when "Hitler sent him to China," when "the world was no longer a pretty place for young people who understood where Hitlerism was leading it," and when the Japanese appeared to be "going in the same direction" that "threatened to take Chiang Kai-shek . . . with them."[51] Like so many of the volunteers in Spain, opposition to Fascism as embodied by Hitler, motivated their professional activism and political affiliations. In 1936, Mao appointed Hatem "Medical Advisor to the Army Department of Health."[52] Hatem became, in the words of biographer Sidney Shapiro, a "superb diplomat without portfolio."[53]

The CAC also used their share of the UCR budget to help fund the travel from Spain to China of a number of refugee doctors from central and Eastern Europe.[54] Nearly two dozen physicians left Spain for China in continuation of the medical work they had begun in Spain.[55] Great Britain's China Medical Aid Committee and a parallel organization in Norway sent others. Most of these physicians were of German or Eastern European origin, and two later wrote memoirs of their experiences.[56] In 1943, at the request of General Joseph Stilwell, some of these physicians were sent to Burma by the Chinese Red Cross to help improve the organization of medical services under the new American command of Chinese forces in the China-Burma theater.

Dr. Hans Mueller was a refugee doctor. Writing in the American magazine *Reader's Scope* in 1945, he offered American readers a glimpse into wartime medical conditions in China through the story of a "typical" Chinese patient. Emphasizing Li's humanity and humility in contrast to the brutality of his Japanese aggressors, Mueller made a case for the needs of the International Peace Hospitals serving patients such as Li. Facing an area of service of six hundred thousand square miles with a population of over 50 million people, Mueller highlighted the enormous medical challenges of the region.[57] Mueller concluded on a positive note, referencing the impact already made by international efforts through people such as Norman Bethune and Dr.

Dwarkanath Kotnis. Kotnis, of the Indian National Congress Medical Mission to China, became director of the West Hopei Hospital before contracting a fatal case of pneumonia.[58] Both Kotnis and Bethune became martyrs to the Chinese cause. Working with the Chinese Eighth Route Army, Bethune cut his finger during a routine operation, contracted sepsis, and died in 1939. He became a legend in China, and to this day the Bethune International Peace Hospital in Shijiazhuang memorializes his name.

The International Peace Hospitals were important destinations for CAC funding. Initiated in July 1938 by the International Peace Campaign's Paris Conference, the International Peace Hospitals initially found their greatest support from the China Campaign Committee in Great Britain.[59] Disrupted by the outbreak of war in Europe, however, the newly formed, China-based, China Defence League helped organize money for the International Peace Hospitals from the U.S., Canada, and New Zealand. The China Defence League (CDL) became the CAC's sister organization in China, distributing the bulk of funds collected by the CAC.

The China Defence League

In 1938, Soong Ching Ling—wife of former Chinese revolutionary Sun Yatsen—helped found the CDL. Conceived of by Soong and Zhou Enlai to organize relief for the armed forces and civilians in the Northwest, the CDL sought to consolidate the anti-Japanese United Front and publicize the efforts of Communist forces against the Japanese.[60] The CDL also sought to connect with foreign groups dedicated to aiding China. Although Soong served as nucleus of the CDL, the organization involved a more international network of people from its inception.[61] James Bertram, a journalist from New Zealand who had spent time with the Eighth Route Army, was an early participant, reporting to Soong Ching Ling the needs of the Chinese wounded from Wuhan.[62] Bertram suggested inviting Mrs. Hilda Selwyn-Clarke, the influential wife of the head of medical services in Hong Kong, to join the league as honorary secretary. One of the group's earliest meetings took place at the home of M.C. Tang, a Cambridge-educated progressive who worked in a Belgian bank, and became one of the league's treasurers, alongside Norman France, a Chinese-born, British professor at Hong Kong University.[63]

The CDL was unequivocal about the hoped-for political ramification of its programs. Soong's assessment of the organization was frank in recognizing its dual purposes in "not just humanitarian relief" but also as a means "to serve the Chinese people's resistance."[64] The CDL, as with the ABMAC and even the AMBASD in Spain, offered clear opposition to idealized traditions of aid emphasizing neutrality above all. Although these groups selectively employed the language of neutrality as a fundraising tool, they emphasized their role as voluntary paramilitary organizations within the conflict in other settings. As echoed in a 1939 report, "The China Defence League is not neutral. Everywhere it helps China's fight. Though its function is purely relief, it applies that relief where it will strengthen the Chinese people in their struggle."[65] Relief, here, was not neutral, and it sought to go beyond compensating for the differences between two sides of a conflict.

In its plan for expanding work in the U.S., the CDL sought to actively focus on promoting its cause among U.S. labor groups. "Committees who aided Spain" were also targeted, and the CDL aimed to "get a group of American doctors to support actively a hospital unit of the International Peace Hospital." It also sought to fundraise for an orthopedic hospital, in cooperation with the ABMAC. Military forces became important targets for CDL aid—particularly the New Fourth Army Medical Bureau and Yenan Base Hospital, whose importance was emphasized to potential private donors for their lack of governmental support.

The "Experts" of UCR

In place of a large volunteer movement of medical personnel, the placement of organizational representatives and logistical liaisons in China was more consistent across the ABMAC, CAC, and UCR. For the ABMAC, Dr. George Bachman served as a salaried ABMAC employee.[66] Dwight W. Edwards filled a parallel role as UCR's field director and representative in China.[67] Edwards had a long history of experience in China. Born in Minnesota and educated at Princeton, Edwards joined the YMCA after completing his masters in mathematics to teach overseas. After one year in Japan, Edwards moved to China, where he spent the next four decades, working for the YMCA, Princeton-in-Peking, Yenching University (a Princeton affiliate), and UCR. Eventually, Edwards focused exclusively on UCR activities, until his retirement and return to the U.S. in 1946.[68] Edwards's assessment of aid recipients was influential in the distribution of UCR funds. He also helped coordinate the diverse array of American private and state organizations active in China the early 1940s.

The ABMAC also drew heavily from Chinese personnel for logistical and representative support. Traveling to Rangoon and Calcutta in March 1942,

Cheng Pao-Nan sent updates to ABMAC leadership on the status of supplies and facilitated the purchase of additional supplies.[69] Szeming Sze also traveled to China in the fall of that year as one of the ABMAC's directors.[70] Still, in its identity as an American institution, the ABMAC did not escape charges of over-involvement in Chinese affairs. In 1943, UCR's Dwight Edwards and Lennig Sweet discussed criticism from some leading Chinese doctors over the "close supervision" that ABMAC had given to some of the projects initiated by Dr. P. Z. King, director of China's National Health Administration.[71] Dr. Marion Yang, however, remained in support of UCR and was "doing her best to put the idea that we are trying to dominate out of the minds of the Chinese people."[72]

The conscious inclusion of Chinese personnel was a departure from pre-existing traditions of sending "expert" Americans to China. In September 1942, Haldore Hanson of the U.S. State Department contacted the ABMAC for assistance in the selection of some such experts. "His request," however, ran "counter to the advice by Dr. Bachman, Dr. King, Dr. Sze and others to send Chinese trained in the methods of Western science, instead of American."[73] The tradition of sending American expertise to China had its roots in the late eighteenth and early nineteenth centuries. Even more recently, the U.S. Division of Cultural Relations had spearheaded similar projects on behalf of the U.S. State Department.

Founded in 1938, the Division of Cultural Relations was established to coordinate international activities in educational and intellectual exchanges in fields of art, music, literature, and other cultural enterprises.[74] The institution also included experts in the fields of medicine and public health as cultural representatives. As remembered by Roger S. Greene, an American diplomat who became involved in China aid through the China Medical Board and American Committee for Non-Participation in Japanese Aggression, the China Section initiated communication with the Chinese government to see if a mission of American expertise would be welcomed. Greene became a consultant to the Division of Cultural Relations, preparing a detailed report in 1942 summarizing the medical situation in China and extent of U.S. aid. Greene highly recommended the inclusion of state-supported cultural exchanges in the medical field, not only for supporting the development of "inductive science" in China, but also because "effective aid to medicine and public health in China should contribute to our victory" in the war.[75]

One of the ways the cultural division explored supporting Greene's recommendations was through sending U.S. medical experts to China. In 1942, Greene presented a list of former medical missionaries who might be willing to return to China under state auspices.[76] Greene suggested that such volunteers might find posts working with the Chinese forces operating under General Stilwell. Between 1941 and 1943, funding for twenty-nine individuals was secured, which included (as decided by the Executive Yuan) experts in medicine and public health, agriculture, and communications.[77] However, with the competing demands of the armed forces and war industries, such experts proved increasingly difficult to find. The State Department found more willing volunteers in recent European immigrants, displaced by the war. Dr. Isidore Snapper, a Dutch citizen in the process of becoming naturalized in the U.S., had the additional support of the China Medical Board for having already served at the PUMC.[78] Another initially promising volunteer (and Austrian immigrant) was rejected for having too strong of a German accent.[79] Regardless of national origin, such volunteers were still considered representatives of the U.S.

As the State Department debated private American medical aid to Spain, the U.S. government increasingly saw medical aid to China as a means of supporting a military ally. Even before U.S. entry into World War II, the U.S. Public Health Service sent a medical commission of experts in malaria prevention to help in the (ultimately failed) construction project of the Yunan-Burma railroad.[80] UCR programs became an opportunity to reinforce state interests in the private sphere, both as a logistical method to maintain sufficient manpower, and as a way to encourage public support in both China and the U.S. of cooperative ventures. Despite being a part of this framework, UCR officials also sought to maintain some distance with state affiliations. For instance, in 1945, the Chinese government offered UCR office space from which to work. Sweet declined the offer, noting that since "UCR is not a military or diplomatic organization and we feel that it would not be justified or wise for us to make use of the kind offices of the Chinese government to provide us with quarters under the regulations for the requisitioning of property," hoping to keep it more firmly within the bounds of civilian and nongovernmental authority.[81] However, the more partisan interests of the ABMAC and the CAC did not always agree with this approach.

The Blockade to the Northwest

The tension between UCR, the ABMAC, and the CAC became particularly pronounced in debates between field personnel of the three organizations over the blockade of Northwest China, which challenged the transmission of funds and supplies. Just as differences of opinion between Nationalist and

Communist forces in China threatened the tentative alliance of the United Front, tensions between the contrasting political allegiances of the ABMAC and the CAC threatened the alliance of UCR. And as relations between Chinese Nationalist sand Chinese Communists deteriorated, so too did the relationships between the ABMAC and CAC within UCR.

Initiated by Nationalist forces to cut off the Japanese in the Northwest, the blockade was equally detrimental to the Chinese Communist forces in the region. Writing to UCR in 1941, the CAC's Forkner discussed the urgency of the situation, attributing the blockade to the intransience of local authorities.[82] With local authorities confiscating goods and materials, American aid organizations found maintaining accountability a problem, as they could no longer insure that goods donated to the region would reach their intended destination. As a result, according to the ABMAC's Bachman, "practically no supplies have been sent to the guerrilla areas" and "it is difficult to get money into the guerrilla areas" as "banks are not willing to take the risk."[83] Additionally, Bachman wrote, "I have been told that the central government is not in favor of sending anything into the guerrilla areas unless there is every assurance that they arrive in the proper hands, and this is difficult to do at the present."[84]

The conditions of the blockade extended to the transmission of information. Still UCR sought ways to assess the situation in the Northwest. When Robert Barnett, liaison officer for UCR, traveled to China, he was given coded instructions by an unknown person in the CAC for ways he could report back on activities in the Northwest. From the simple telegram, "ARRIVED CHUNGKING SAFE HEALTH EXCELLENT," Barnett would provide the telegram recipient with a detailed account of the status of Mme. Sun's programs. "ARRIVED," Barnett was instructed, was to mean that he had seen Mme. Sun and talked to her about medical aid. "CHUNGKING" was to indicate that the guerrilla areas were no longer being blockaded (with its omission from the telegram indicating the opposite). "SAFE" or "SAFELY" was to indicate that money could safely be sent to the peace hospitals. If "IS" was added to "HEALTH EXCELLENT," Barnett could communicate there had been specific news from the hospital in North Kiangsu regarding a recent transmission of supplies.

In 1943, UCR's Edwards advised against accepting gifts designated for the Northwest as a logistical impossibility. While "we are all very sympathetic informally . . . it is generally agreed that any request for priority to ship medical supplies designated for this purpose into China would not only meet with flat refusal but also prejudice those making the request in the eyes of the authorities," with the problem being "not so much a lack of supplies as it is the transport of supplies."[85] As evidence, Edwards reported the failure of two trucks of supplies sent two years prior to reach their destination after being detained by local authorities. The question of the blockade had already been a matter of discussion for Edwards and Sweet. The year before, Sweet had noted in communication with Edwards, "Many of us over here feel that it is not fair that there should be practically an embargo against them and that strong pressure should be put on to suggest to the Chinese Government that they be given money and supplies which have been forwarded from this country."[86] Edwards was more reticent. Responding a few months later, Edwards summarized his views on UCR donations to the Eighth Route Army in the Northwest, particularly as channeled through the CAC:

> The political tension is such that the committee of ours, which in its personnel and particularly in its Chairman, has those who are in political life, will find it very difficult to discuss this question and to reach any judgment which is well balanced and unbiased. By this I do not mean that they personally would not approve of helping in this region; but the knowledge that they were participating in aid to these people would be used against them politically and might even involve their personal freedom. I think that their own committee will have to be content with what recommendation I send personally to them in this connection. Of course I will act in full consultation with the CDL and shall try to obtain as unbiased a view point as possible. However, I hesitate very much to bring this question up for any formal discussion.[87]

By Edwards's assessment, the political overtones inherent in aid to the Northwest, particularly in supplies directed explicitly to Communist military forces, put UCR's ability to work in other parts of China at risk. Operating, as it did, with the approval and cooperation of the Nationalist government, Edwards did not hesitate in implying that involvement in CAC activities could pose a risk to UCR.

Edwards had also taken a highly critical view toward Lim and the Emergency Medical Service Training Schools (EMSTS) of the CRC—a high priority for the ABMAC. His assessment contributed to sparking an open battle between ABMAC and UCR leadership, which had as much to do with ongoing disagreements over decision-making in program operations and financial appropriations.[88] While his criticism rested primarily on reports of corruption and inefficiency among the EMSTS, led by Lim, he also openly questioned the ABMAC's emphasis on medical aid directed toward military endeavors. Such attitudes placed him opposite those of UCR's Medical Committee, particularly those of the Army Medical Sub-Committee.[89] Dominated by the ABMAC, UCR's Medical Committee included all seventeen members of the ABMAC Medical Committee, with Helen Kennedy Stevens of the ABMAC acting as secretary.[90] The ABMAC's Co Tui chaired the group's military subcommittee and argued strongly for army medical aid as central to China's resistance and therefore of high priority to ABMAC and UCR aid—an opinion that became one shared by the committee as a whole.[91] Forkner, for instance, as another member of this sub-committee, reported being "amazed to find that the recommendations of the medical subcommittee of UCR (ABMAC Committee) were largely disregarded by Edwards's committee."[92]

This conflict turned into one of structural significance, with ABMAC questioning Edwards's presence in China and role in managing an office abroad, and CAC representatives supporting his assessments and foreign position. The CAC's Alice Carter defended Edwards's position with a comparison to the ARC's processes in noting that, "In employing a field director, UCR is using the same procedure as the ARC which has its representatives all over the world."[93] The controversy surrounding Edwards's recommendation surrounding the EMSTS became a question of the appropriate role of the agency in administering relief abroad. The CAC and UCR pushed for the proactive presence of American representatives (by the standards set by the ARC) with some independence of action, while the ABMAC sought a closer and more exclusive relationship with Chinese Nationalist authorities. While the ABMAC supported a proposal for the chairman of the UCR Program Committee in China to be appointed by the Executive Yuan itself, the CAC sided with UCR leadership in the concern that such an action would "endanger . . . the whole American concept of administering relief through private agencies free from government influence."[94] In these debates, CAC leadership emphasized its role within UCR as a humanitarian organization seeking discerning judgment in the efficiency and neutrality of destined recipients of UCR aid.

However, at the same time, the question of the blockade remained, for the CAC, a matter of equal importance by the same discerning standards. Encouraged by reports from the CDL, lifting the blockade became a matter of humanitarian necessity. Writing to CAC executive director Mildred Price in

1943 of recent resolutions made for cooperation between the Nationalists and Communists, Soong Ching Ling suggested that such resolutions gave "good ground for an immediate campaign in America for the *lifting of the blockade* at least on medical supplies" as, "if equality of all parties is promised after the war," it was "obviously high time that the equality of wounded fighters in their right to medication and treatment should be made real *immediately*."[95] Soong argued passionately, "The grotesque anomaly of this situation should be resolved at once, and in our favor. It is time to mobilize relief organizations and people of good will in America for this non-partisan objective, and to make it a *test* of our government's professions of tolerance and democratic aspirations."[96] Soong's argument reveals the common expectation of many of these private organizations to stimulate state action.

The blockade was eventually relaxed with regard to the transport of medical supplies. In 1944, the U.S. ambassador to China reported to the secretary of state that the central government had begun allowing selective passage of medical aid. He attributed the change to pressure arising from publicity given to a message from Soong Ching Ling in an unspecified American publication and increasing attention from foreign press correspondents.[97] As reported in January 1945, ten tons of supplies had been marked for movement from Yunnan province to Yenan for the International Peace Hospitals.[98] With over five tons already moved by the U.S. Army, the ARC noted that publicity over this shipment had to be kept quiet until the army completed its mission. Ultimately, the ARC and U.S. Army proved essential in orchestrating the logistics.

Private Aid and State Responsibility

As much as Edwards provided an important link for UCR in China, he had also become a point of controversy. Differences between headquarters and field offices might be expected in any organization, particularly those spanning large geographical distances. But how much of this controversy was as much a result of the dualism between state and voluntary impulses within UCR? These battles evidenced more fundamental disagreements in what relative roles various private and state efforts should assume. The ABMAC's affiliations sought to build an intimate relationship with Nationalist health structures—cooperating closely with Chinese officials in the National Health Administration, Army Medical Services, and Chinese Red Cross Society. Meanwhile, the CAC argued against an overly intimate relationship with Nationalist leaders, emphasizing UCR's responsibility as a private organization to act independently of government structures, while also serving CAC interests in sending aid to areas outside of Nationalist control. At the same time, the CAC maintained close ties to another private organization in China working in close collaboration with Chinese Communist groups. For the ABMAC, the CAC and Chinese Communists comprised a real political threat, just as the ABMAC and Chinese Nationalists did for the CAC.

Edwards framed his criticism and support on what he deemed to be the most efficient application of UCR funds. Given the very real difficulty of getting funds and supplies to the Northwest, supporting more established Nationalist enterprises was argued to be a more practical use of UCR resources. Edwards revealed more of his own perspective by contrasting support of Chinese military medical services with the needs caused by the 1943 Honan famine. Reporting on the famine to Sweet, Edwards noted:

> The situation is very serious, and Kiangsi, Chekiang and Kwangtung all present problems which demand heavy support. It has been argued by some that the Government is responsible for the relief of the people in these stricken districts and particularly Honan. The argument could be applied very much more cogently to the Army Medical Administration. In this case, there is no factor of natural disaster or aggression on the part of the enemy, and it is a proposition, in which the Government is 100% responsible, for which it can provide funds if it so desires and in which it has the support of its Allied friends.[99]

Edwards differentiated the responsibilities of the state in natural versus man-made disasters. Not only did Edwards maintain the expectation that the Chinese government ought to be responsible for the basic medical needs of its own military forces, but he also emphasized the American military's additional responsibility as a military ally of China. Referring again to the debate over the EMSTS, Edwards's perception of state responsibility played a significant role in his criticism of UCR support for Lim's program. Beyond citing noted inefficiencies in the current administration of the EMSTS, Edwards also argued that it was not worth UCR support as other resources—including those of the U.S. Army Medical Service—were available for the same purpose (i.e. the training of military medical personnel). According to communications between Edwards and Colonel Williams of the U.S. Army Medical Service's new training program of Chinese medics, Col. Williams was not only "quite in agreement with the policy of the Committee on Coordination," but welcomed the possibility of UCR support of his program.[100]

Conclusions

The activities of the ABMAC and CAC had not come to be defined by groups of medical volunteers, as the AMBASD had in Spain. The ABMAC and CAC sent limited numbers of medical volunteers, most of Chinese or foreign origin. In contrast to the relative autonomy sought by the AMBASD in action, private U.S. aid organizations in China focused more on supporting Chinese institutions. With that, groups such as the ABMAC, CAC, and UCR faced larger debates over the relative roles of private and public enterprise in aid. Conflicts expressed with UCR and its member organizations that began as disagreements surrounding a particular program transitioned into larger debates and intra-organizational hostility. From this perspective, one must wonder how many individual differences originated in personal factors only framed by larger political issues. Questions of power between Chinese personnel and institutions and U.S. "expertise" within aid organizations challenged the personnel and representatives of UCR. While organizations such as the ABMAC and the CAC found an early advantage in more openly embracing their own political leanings, both were asked to dampen aspects of their own political agendas within the joint effort of UCR. This was a difficult process, often leading to friction between the ABMAC, the CAC, and UCR. And moving from an organizational to an individual level, political dimensions multiply in complexity.

CHAPTER SIX

The Politics of Relief

Just as the organizations of this study were organizations that arose from conflict, they also became organizations that largely disintegrated with the resolution of conflict. As popular responses to the outbreak of war in Spain and in China, the AMBASD, ABMAC, and CAC initially claimed organizational identity in contrast to state and institutional responses. These groups suggested that the moral imperative rested with the American people to respond to and support particular foreign groups in political crisis when the state and other aid institutions failed to respond. But as the Nationalists gained control in Spain, international aid to the Spanish Republic diminished. And as World War II in China gave way to the Chinese Civil War, the combined effort of UCR struggled to remain integrated before eventually dissolving. The ABMAC moved more of its focus to Taiwan, alongside the Nationalist government of China, and the CAC faded into obscurity as Communist China closed its borders to the outside.

Following the end of the Spanish Civil War and Second Sino-Japanese War, the politics of relief for the AMBASD, ABMAC, and CAC became internalized, as infighting grew and the individual members of all faced a different post-war environment for aid in the U.S. Groups such as the AMBASD and CAC confronted allegations over their dealings with foreign Communist groups, and the integrated effort of UCR found itself outpaced by new post-war institutions of aid. With the rise of anti-Communism in the U.S., the ways in which political activism in the 1930s had become intertwined with the provision of medical aid led to accusations of how the partisan relief of these groups had become more of a dangerous subversion to national interests than a humanitarian expression of international ideals.

The Veteran Volunteers of Spain

With the end of the Spanish Civil War, AMBASD volunteers who had been in Spain returned home to face new challenges. A few ambulance drivers who had only recently immigrated to the U.S. before volunteering had difficulty re-entering the U.S. because of visa issues.[1] Many more had difficulties finding work. For some, injuries or illnesses acquired in Spain hampered their attempts to reestablish themselves professionally. The AMBASD offered assistance to some, providing letters of recommendation or other small financial contributions to help pay doctors' bills.[2] For others, attitudes toward the political connotations of having gone to Spain were reported to be the biggest obstacle. Although she eventually found employment in the medical clinic of the Soviet pavilion, Luba Brisker attributed her difficulties in finding work to having been in Spain.[3]

For others, however, their wartime experience in Spain offered a foundation for later service with U.S. military units in World War II. Among AMBASD personnel to serve were nurses Rose Abramson, Ave Bruzzichesi, Selma Chadwick, Fanny Golub, Salaria Kee, Clara Leight, and Hilda Bell Roberts; doctors Abraham Ettelson, Julius Hene, and Sidney Vogel; physical therapist Eugenia Grunsky; and dental technician Joseph Highkin. Rose Weiner volunteered for service with the ARC, U.S. Army, and War Manpower Commission, but was rejected for being "1 inch short and 13 lbs underweight."[4] William Pike became a colonel in the U.S. Army Air Corps.[5] Dentist Jack Klein volunteered, but the U.S. Army's investigation took so long that he became overage for service.[6] Rose Wachsman also volunteered and was reportedly to be sent to Germany, but in the end remained in service in the U.S. because of her "questionable" background.[7] Leo Eloesser volunteered but reported being rejected, according to Eloesser, for "premature anti-fascism."[8] Both Eloesser and Bruzzichesi eventually became part of UN medical services.[9] Helen Freeman worked in Germany as a public health nurse for German refugees from 1947 to 1949.[10] A number of other AMBASD personnel, including Dr. Abraham Friedman, nurse George Moser, and ambulance driver Council Carter, publicly discussed going to China after the war ended.[11]

Back in the U.S., the volunteers of the AMBASD joined surviving members of the Abraham Lincoln Brigade (ALB) in their veteran association—the Veterans of the Abraham Lincoln Brigade (VALB). The VALB offered a common ground for those who shared the experience of the war in Spain and continued to promote the cause of the Spanish Republic while keeping alive the memory of those who participated. On the one hand, this direct alliance between the volunteer combatants of the ALB with the medical volunteers of the AMBASD reinforces the idea that volunteers of both forces served in Spain as part of the same military effort. This connection seems to have led to contemporary accounts that do little to differentiate between the military volunteers of the ALB and the medical volunteers of the AMBASD. While the volunteer movements of the ALB and AMBASD may have become intertwined in Spain, it misses a part of the picture to equate the two entirely. Although there were certainly overlaps in their work and support, the ALB and AMBASD arose as two distinct (albeit related) responses to the Spanish Civil War.

In differentiating or equating these movements historically, political pressures complicate the accounts of AMBASD volunteers. As nurse Fredericka Martin lamented to a friend in 1970: "Most of our former co-laborers in Spain have successfully buried their memories of Spain, almost as if deliberately. I suspect that the pressure of McCarthyism induced this reaction—if questioned they would truly remember. The least political people remember most clearly all sorts of details . . . the most religious members of our units—staunch defenders of their service there—also recall events freely and clearly."[12] The intensity of anti-Communist sentiment in the U.S. in the decades that followed the Spanish Civil War must be taken into account in studying the memories of AMBASD volunteers. And yet, amid those open to speaking of their experience, none regretted his or her decision to go to Spain. In interviews and correspondence from the 1950s onward, AMBASD volunteers express the value of their experience in Spain. As described by Brisker, "In spite of the hardships encountered there, I consider the experience of being in Spain, of trying to help the Spanish people fight fascism one of the most satisfying two years of my life and which brought me the greatest personal benefits in every respect."[13] Even Albert Byrne, who encountered more difficulties than most given his period of imprisonment, later called Spain the "greatest experience I ever had."[14] Others were less effusive, albeit without regret. As expressed briefly when asked if she regretted going to Spain, physical therapist Eugenia Grunsky replied, "No—most miserable and interesting year I ever had."[15]

The challenges of memory in the aftermath of the war not only affected the lives of many volunteers, but also seeped deeply into the historical record. To this day, the Spanish Civil War remains a highly polarized historical chapter. Many volunteers claimed that simply having been in Spain lost them jobs and opportunities. And in the aftermath of the war, many faced legal action or prosecution in relation to their activities in Spain. Not long after its volunteers had returned to the U.S. and the war in Spain had ended, the Medical Bureau and North American Committee to Aid Spanish Democracy attracted the attention of the House Un-American Activities Committee (HUAC).[16] In February of 1940, authorities arrested two doctors of the AMBASD for violation of an 1818 U.S. statute that prohibited the recruitment of Americans in foreign armies.[17] Although both were released and all charges dismissed, the incident became just one of many to affect AMBASD veterans. Such cases directly addressed the question that had fueled State Department debates—whether medical volunteers were to be considered part of a military effort. In doing so, medical aid was identified as a corollary to military intervention, which could turn AMBASD activities into treason. While the intimacy of AMBASD units with Republican army forces might have supported such claims, such laws were also invoked selectively.

Five months after the end of World War II, HUAC issued subpoenas to Barsky and other executives of the Joint Anti-Fascist Refugee Committee (JAFRC). Barsky had helped found the JAFRC in 1941, and within a couple of years the JAFRC had raised nearly $400,000 in support of Spanish refugees while continuing to lobby the U.S. government on behalf of the exiled Republican government. When Barsky and his colleagues refused to submit the organization's financial records and the names of contributors and recipients of aid, they were held in contempt of Congress and convicted in June 1947.[18] After three years of appeals challenging the constitutionality of the HUAC hearings, the Supreme Court refused to review the convictions. Barsky was sentenced to six months in prison and fined $500, while other members of the JAFRC executive board were given lighter penalties. Dr. Louis Miller, who had hosted some of the earliest meetings leading to the formation of the AMBASD, was one of those also involved.[19] In December 1947, the ALB, VALB, and JAFRC were all declared subversive organizations by Attorney General Tom Clark. Following the McCarran Internal Security Act of 1950, the VALB was required to register as an agent of a foreign government. Four years later, the organization faced the Subversive Activity Control Board, which alleged a direct link between the ALB and the Communist Party.

Returning to New York after serving his sentence at the federal penitentiary in Petersburg, Virginia, Barsky faced censure by the New York State Board of Regents, which suspended his medical license because of his conviction. Although many of Barsky's medical colleagues filed an Amicus Curiae on his behalf, after four years of appeals the Supreme Court upheld the six-month suspension. As observed in Judge William O. Douglas's dissenting opinion in 1954, "So far as I know, nothing in a man's political beliefs disables him from setting broken bones or removing ruptured appendixes safely and efficiently . . . When a doctor cannot save lives in America because he is opposed to Franco in Spain, it is time to call a halt and look critically at the neurosis that has possessed us."[20]

Barsky was not the only AMBASD volunteer who reported persecution in the U.S. for his time in Spain. In 1957, nurse Ena Ferwerda was suspended from her job at a Veterans Hospital in Togus, Maine, for her past "subversive" activities.[21] She was granted a hearing after a few months, at which she showed her passport, stamped "valid for Spain."[22] Ferwerda won her case and was re-instated at the hospital eight months later, with back pay. In Florida, nurse Rose Wachsman received a court subpoena for activities relating to her time in Spain—which had already been reported as the reason she was fired from a prior job in New York.[23] When nurse Lini De Vries began receiving visits from the FBI, she decided that "the future looked decidedly bleak" and moved to Mexico.[24] Martin, also seeking a different political climate, moved to Mexico in the 1950s.[25]

In contrast to the AMBASD and American participants in the International Brigades, not only did the similarly partisan ABMAC and CAC find U.S. support through UCR, but the American Volunteer Group (AVG) also created a private military outlet for Americans seeking to support Nationalist China and gain combat experience before U.S. entry into the war. The "Flying Tigers," as the AVG was also known, were a group of American pilots who volunteered to serve alongside nascent Chinese air forces and the British Royal Air Force in Burma. Formed at the request of Chiang Kai-shek and his wife, and organized in the U.S. by retired American colonel Claire Lee Chennault, the AVG saw action in China for less than a year before the unit was absorbed into the U.S. Army Air Force as the 23rd Fighter Group. To work within U.S. neutrality legislation, the AVG operated through private institutions, allowing the U.S. to maintain formally neutral relations with Japan.[26] As Madame Chiang Kai-shek confided in a letter to Helen Kennedy Stevens of the ABMAC, "Before Pearl Harbor, the only two forces which convinced the Chinese people that Americans were fond of them and concerned about their welfare were General Claire L. Chennault's Flying Tigers and ABMAC."[27] In contrast, several U.S. pilots who traveled to Spain to offer air support to the Republican government were later investigated by the U.S. Attorney's office for violation of the statute prohibiting enlistment in foreign armies—the same statute that was suggested as a basis for the possible subpoena of the AMBASD first unit of medical volunteers.[28]

Although noteworthy parallels between the wars in China and Spain exist, the political dimensions of each opened very different avenues of U.S. involvement. But there were still overlaps. Among AMBASD volunteers who sought service with U.S. armed forces in World War II, the majority was able to put wartime experience to use. This was not the case for all, nor did this acceptance extend unchallenged in the years after the war. Perhaps, in this light, the arguments for the "myth" of "premature antifascism" warrant consideration.[29] To do so does not have to negate or condone the challenges faced by so many volunteers after the war, but does perhaps shift the terms under which we continue to discuss the aftermath of veteran involvement in the decades that followed.

"United" China Relief

The force of anti-Communism in the U.S. also affected UCR organizations such as the CAC, although less is known about the extent to which this may have affected personnel involved. Without a volunteer base of comparable size to that of the AMBASD, the CAC may not have felt quite the same impact, despite the fact that HUAC also listed the group as a subversive organization.[30] Even before, in the early days of UCR, the CAC posed a challenge to the unified aid effort UCR proposed. As described by the ABMAC's Frank Co Tui in 1939:

> It is almost impossible for the newly created organizations to merge. The China Aid Council . . . is identified in the eyes of the majority of Americans as leftists and even communistic. This is not wholly true but the impression is there. To have China's cause identified with leftism in the eyes of America would be suicidal . . . The Bureau [ABMAC] must not only dissociate itself from the China Aid Council but must take the leadership in the relief field. The statement has been made that to differentiate between right and left here when there is union in China is divisive tactics. But it is precisely because of our effort to present a picture of democratic unity that we must not allow recognized leftists in America to dominate the picture in Chinese relief work.[31]

Co Tui framed the problems of the CAC's political orientation in light of a failing campaign of aid to Spain, while also emphasizing his own strategic interpretation of the American political climate. Preceding the founding of HUAC by several years, Co Tui's comments and perceptions of U.S. attitudes toward Communism would prove prescient. When the United Front alliance between the Kuomintang and Chinese Communist Party disintegrated back into the Chinese Civil War in the latter half of the 1940s, UCR struggled to maintain a sense of shared purpose as members within these organizations became more deeply entrenched in their political differences.

UCR's parallel fragmentation centered on the CAC and relief efforts in the northwest of China, the principal territory of the Chinese Communists. Edwards wrote to the UCR chairman in the fall of 1945, urging a reconsideration of UCR support of the China Defence League (which received money through the CAC) in light of the acceleration of civil war in China. Sweet agreed that the matter ought to be reviewed, with the qualification that "a very strong minority in our constituency would be very angry if we did not continue to support the Northwest program, while others are insistent that none of their money go to Chinese communists." By Sweet's estimate, the programs in question received about 5 percent of UCR funds ($104,000). Not only was the figure a relatively small portion of the UCR budget, but it was also only a fraction of other aid reaching China Defence League programs from abroad. The Canadian government was reportedly sending $650,000, with the Canadian ambassador demonstrating a personal interest in the International Peace Hospitals, "motivated . . . by a desire to use Canadian funds in such a way as to be a predominantly Canadian supported project and thus bring Canada's name before the Chinese public."[32]

In October of 1946, a man named Alfred Kohlberg wrote to UCR officials on behalf of the American China Policy Association demanding evidence that UCR funds channeled through the CAC to the CDL had reached their intended destination for their intended purpose: medical aid.[33] Kohlberg alleged that he suspected that some part of the $715,737.52 in question had been "diverted for purposes of Communist propaganda."[34] While Kohlberg conceded the value, generally speaking, of "non-partisanship in relief," his demands were framed in opposition to the practice of extending aid to "allies and enemies alike."[35] For Kohlberg, the political significance of relief seemed to outweigh any humanitarian intentions. And, in the case of China, the Communists were the primary enemy for Kohlberg. "We have info," Kohlberg wrote, "that the money does not go to the ostensible objectives of the charity, but is turned over for the use of the Communist underground in Nationalist China."[36] As evidence Kohlberg highlighted that UCR funds were channeled to the CDL in U.S. dollars and Chinese yen—neither of which, according to Kohlberg, were valid forms of currency in Communist regions.

In the months that followed, UCR continued to send funds to the Northwest as Kohlberg's letters went unanswered. However, debates over the CAC remained, and when supplies to the International Peace Hospitals appeared to be held up, CAC leadership became suspicious of UCR's ongoing support. Sweet seemed to dismiss such suspicions without much concern. Reporting the matter to Edwards he wrote, "I am quite sure this is entirely without foundation," while also noting that, "in view of all the tensions, we must lean over backwards to not even seem to be prejudiced."[37] Sweet went on to suggest that the CAC's strong and clearly defined political motivations were becoming a hindrance to the organization's real work and purpose. What had been a strength for the group before the war seemed to have become a liability in the postwar political climate.

As the constituent groups of UCR showed increasing political polarization, UCR officials tried to adjust the responsibilities and fields of expertise of each to minimize conflict. By Edwards's ideal, the ABMAC was to take charge of the field of medical relief—without "centering its interest on national medicine and public health"—while the CAC's passions were to be neutralized by giving the group "broader responsibilities so that objectivity becomes necessary."[38] Although the ABMAC had, by this time, become increasingly focused on medical education, its funds were still heavily bent toward government medical schools. Considering the possibility of granting the CAC leadership in the field of child welfare under UCR, Sweet concluded, "They are such outstanding proponents of the work in the communist areas, there will be great danger that they would be involved in such a complex of political, medical and child welfare programs that much confusion would be added to the picture."[39] By July 1947, the majority of the $800,000 budgeted to child welfare was associated with the CAC.[40]

In 1948, UCR's medical program continued to support a broad range of programs, including 150 Protestant and Catholic mission hospitals, private hospitals through the American Advisory Committee, International Peace Hospitals through the CAC, and government projects through the ABMAC.[41] International Peace Hospital support included ten hospitals, consisting of eight thousand beds, which offered free service to patients and some medical training. These hospitals covered an area serving 140 million people. The private hospital support offered by the American Advisory Committee was principally in transporting medical supplies and offering training subsidies, serving nearly five hundred dispensaries and clinics, which included Chinese, Catholic, and Protestant institutions. The ABMAC was working to support students through the Chinese Medical Association, in addition to promoting medical education through a fellowship program and providing equipment for eleven teaching institutions. It was also still involved in the pyrogen-free fluid and blood bank projects.[42]

By this time, Alfred Kohlberg had gained a reputation among UCR leadership for his zealotry, and threats to make his accusations against the CAC public appeared to reinforce this attitude. UCR records suggest that most of his letters went unanswered, although internal communication indicates that discussions were held regarding the need for investigation of CAC funds to the China Defence League. Throughout most of this episode, UCR leadership's primary concern seemed to be the avoidance of the negative publicity that might arise from more public accusations, especially at a time when the organization was already struggling with a postwar decline in fundraising. It is unclear how exactly this conflict was resolved, but eventually Kohlberg's missives faded out of UCR's records of communication. Perhaps the CAC's recordkeeping had maintained sufficient evidence that the nearly $1.5 million it channeled to medical projects in the Northwest reached its intended destination. If it did, this was not reported in UCR's saved correspondence with Kohlberg. The limited UCR response to Kohlberg's latest wave of allegations does, at least, seem to suggest that he was not considered a significant figure.

In the end, the CAC was never indicted by UCR officials, nor does any substantial evidence appear in UCR financial records to suggest that CAC funds were being used for anything other than their intended purposes in medical and child welfare. Some of the individuals involved, however, faced personal allegations over their political views, similar to those experienced by AMBASD volunteers returning from Spain. Both Mildred Price (executive secretary of the CAC) and Duncan Lee (on the CAC's Executive Board) have been identified in some research as active agents in Soviet espionage.[43] Meanwhile, Philip Jaffe, editor of the journal *Amerasia* and one of those charged with illegal possession of confidential government documents in the *Amerasia* affair, was also a CAC board member, and later the organization's treasurer. Edward C. Carter, another target of Kohlberg's in connection to *Amerasia* was involved in UCR. His wife, Alice Carter, served among CAC leadership. Supporting at least a distrust of Nationalist China, UCR records suggest that, "Mrs. Carter . . . does not wish CAC to be too closely tied up with any movement of the central government and I think if CAC support is to be given, she will have to be assured that there will be no government domination of the program."[44]

Further details about Price are difficult to find. In June 1942, Price accepted an invitation from Carter to join the UCR Program Committee.[45] Four years later, she traveled to China on behalf of her work with the CAC and UCR, with the intention of spending up to six months abroad. Briefing Edwards on her expected arrival via UNRRA plane in May, Sweet reported to Edwards that Price was in China to organize a China-based committee for the CAC, based on the rationale that if ABMAC had such a committee, the CAC should have one too. Sweet encouraged Edwards to involve her as much as possible in providing the tools to more effectively review UCR's child welfare budget and work. From UCR's perspective, "The real purpose of the trip is to help Mildred Price become more effective after her return rather than to give any special technical assistance at present."[46]

Alfred Kohlberg

While perhaps exceptional in the extent of his activism, Alfred Kohlberg, a businessman, passionate sinophile, and vigorous anti-Communist, in many ways offers an interesting example of the ways in which political activism of this period and these organizations became expressed through the foundation and work of the organizations themselves. By the early 1940s, Kohlberg had begun searching for a philanthropic outlet to supplement his commercial engagements in China. Investigating American aid agencies operating in China, the ABMAC earned Kohlberg's approval in both prioritizing Chinese interests and keeping overhead costs low. As Kohlberg's involvement deepened, he joined the organization's board of directors and traveled to China (on personal funds) a number of times to report on ABMAC's field programs in operation.

From participation in private American aid to China through the ABMAC, by 1943 Kohlberg had been contacted by representatives of both the Chinese and U.S. governments regarding his work. In March of that year, J. Heng Liu, public health officer with the Nationalist government, wrote to Kohlberg suggesting that AMBAC and UCR representatives Bachman and Greene were "grossly misinformed" about the financial backing for medical supplies to the Chinese army, and were falsely perpetuating the "impression that the Chinese Army Medical Service and the Public Health Service are entirely supported, in cash as well as in supplies from American sources."[47] Around the same time, Roosevelt's Far East advisor, Lauchlin Currie, summoned Kohlberg to Washington D.C. to express concerns over reports of the "hopelessness" of the Chinese National government and its armies.[48] Both Liu and Currie seemed to identify Kohlberg as a potential resource based on his extensive involvement in China for both business and private aid.

Kohlberg seemed to take these connections seriously, and when he returned to China in the summer of 1943, he sought to investigate rumors that supplies being sent to the Chinese Red Cross from the U.S. were ending up on the black market instead. During this trip, Kohlberg visited Chinese forces on Ninth War Front, traveling through five provinces against the recommendations of American officials and without the typically required permits.[49] Returning from these travels, Kohlberg concluded that all charges against the Chinese were "totally untrue or substantially exaggerated."[50] Although Kohlberg found that sulfa drugs were being sold on the black market after being sneaked over the hump, he discovered no ABMAC supplies implicated in these transactions. What became a greater concern for Kohlberg was the fact that his observations of a competent and dedicated Nationalist army did not correspond with the reports he had become privy to in Washington. This trip marked the beginning of a vocal campaign by Kohlberg on behalf of Chiang Kai-shek's Nationalist government.

After his 1943 trip, Kohlberg also began to question UCR's involvement in China. Kohlberg's criticism of UCR came on multiple levels: its basic inefficiency and irrelevance as an organization since the development of the National War Fund, its failure to provide sufficient emphasis on army medical aid, its placement of Dwight W. Edwards in the position of field representative, and its alleged "missionary bias."[51] Kohlberg blamed Edwards (and ABMAC representative George Bachman) for Robert Lim's ejection from leadership of the Chinese Red Cross and the separation of the Chinese Red Cross and EMSTS.[52] When the UCR board investigated Kohlberg's charges against Edwards, he was exonerated from all.[53] The result led Kohlberg to accuse UCR of being insensitive to China's real needs. By Kohlberg's analysis, there were two principal communities in China seeking UCR support: the foreign groups with missionary ties and the newly developed institutions of the Chinese government and military.[54] Kohlberg noted that in drawing predominantly from the American missionary community for staffing, Chinese leaders and institutions suspected UCR of unjust partiality. In Kohlberg's own dramatic words, "Criticism of China and Chinese institutions by missionaries, among themselves, to other Americans, to American military personnel and in reports home, all of which eventually comes back to Chinese ears, is building up to a crescendo of misunderstanding, with results that I fear to contemplate."[55] When the ABMAC refused to withdraw from UCR, Kohlberg resigned as chairman of the ABMAC Executive Committee and ABMAC director.[56]

For Kohlberg, like many others of this study, organizations were key to the expression of his political beliefs. His associations and resignations illustrated not only the evolution of his political beliefs, but also the patterns of his expectations of organizational action. From his interest in Asia and participation in the board of the Institute of Pacific Relations, Kohlberg resigned from the board and initiated a personal battle against the institution when he decided it had become infiltrated by Communist interests seeking to undermine the Nationalist Chinese government.[57] Kohlberg's activism helped generate one of the first legal cases of Cold War espionage in "the Amerasia affair."[58] After withdrawing his support from the ABMAC and UCR, Kohlberg went on to help found the American China Policy Association in 1946 and the American Jewish League against Communism in 1948.[59] In short, organizations became the currency of Kohlberg's political life as a private citizen—a currency shared by many of the individuals behind the wave of private action in the U.S. in the late 1930s and early 1940s.

UCR and the New Institutions of Aid

During the war, however, the landscape of American relief had begun to change. Founded in 1943, the United Nations Relief and Rehabilitation Administration (UNRRA) claimed to offer a new form of international relief work, having begun planning toward postwar relief and reconstruction as early as 1941.[60] Under predominantly U.S. leadership, UNRRA's greatest interests remained focused around the needs of central-eastern Europe. In China, however, UCR became involved in distributing a significant amount of UNRRA materials and supplies. Their work in this realm reportedly earned UCR an unsolicited commendation from UNRRA, which "hoped that during the coming year some similar arrangement can be evolved for handling a percentage of the post-UNRRA relief which the American people are to send to China through Congressional grants."[61] Other organizations, such as the Chinese Nation Relief and Rehabilitation Administration (CNRRA) and China Liberated Areas Relief Association (CLARA), were also operating as conduits of aid from other sources, with a primary focus on the International Peace Hospitals, although working broadly across the areas liberated from Japanese control.[62] In 1946, however, the UNRRA dissolved, making way for the United Nations and its specialized organizations.

That same year also saw the dissolution of the National War Fund, followed by the foundation of a new national federation for foreign services in the U.S., American Overseas Aid (AOA). Since the National War Fund had been liquidated, the major foreign aid agencies that had fallen under its jurisdiction had once again been left to independent fundraising campaigns, a change that reportedly created greater competition, confusion, and public hostility to foreign relief. After the supposed failure of many campaigns in

1947, the AOA sought to return to earlier models, streamlining such requests into a single appeal. Despite its official-sounding pedigree, the AOA, it was argued, was "in essence a People's Movement," offering a channel through which "the goodwill and generosity of the American people may be expressed" as "a dramatic demonstration of the typical American spirit to participate voluntarily in the relief of human needs and to promote human welfare."[63] The AOA was to take responsibility for raising UCR's 1948 funds.[64] At the same time, UCR publicity emphasized the qualities that set it apart from the newly developing government organizations. As a "private, personalized effort," UCR had the potential to "be a catalyst to hasten the series of reactions which will make China a modern, democratic nation."[65] UCR argued that its status as a private organization freed it from bureaucratic red tape, enabling it to act more swiftly and efficiently than government programs, with lower administrative costs.[66]

Even as the AOA emphasized the program's popular foundation, many of its fundraising appeals were crafted for the American corporate community. For decades, American philanthropy had been funded and, in large part, defined by America's corporate bodies. In marketing its fundraising activities to corporate donors, the AOA recognized this role even more explicitly:

> American business certainly didn't create the problems which beset most of the overseas world, but American business cannot hope to escape their depressing effects. You don't have to be in the export trade to know that all American enterprise has something vitally important at stake in what is happening on the other sides of the oceans which surround us. The U.S. Government is moving in official channels to extend basic assistance to foreign nations whose economic well-being is vital to our own stability. Is government economic assistance enough?[67]

Corporations were encouraged to consider themselves as extensions of the government, with a shared interest in U.S. state interests. "Corporations, as legal entities," AOA publicity suggested, "are creatures of government, and government recognizes the obligation of corporations to make gifts to philanthropic causes by providing a legal income tax deduction for such gifts . . . as a necessary and essential part of our foreign aid policy."[68] President Truman himself offered a letter of endorsement.[69]

In 1949, as the civil war in China reached its climax, UCR produced a detailed policy statement delineating its purpose. This statement offered an argument as to why individual Americans should feel a responsibility beyond government initiatives for offering assistance to China. In this, Chinese and American interests were directly linked, in ways that make the document look as much like a foreign policy statement as a philosophy of humanitarian aid.[70] Through its emphasis on the larger geopolitical ramifications of offering assistance to China, the proffered aid almost appeared to take a place secondary to interests of foreign relations. China's value to U.S. interests lay in its perceived position as a critical component to the balance of power in Asia, particularly in light of the rising conflict between Communist and democratic nations. UCR's policy statement stuck closely to the American narrative of a unique Sino-American friendship. As part of this tradition, UCR argued, "We enjoy their respect and trust because they like our free form of government, the basic philosophy of our people and the proven sincerity of our non-imperialistic international policy."[71] UCR also cited China and America's long history of educational and business exchanges in suggesting that China now looked to the U.S. for guidance. Risk was involved in that "if we do not take advantage of this opportunity to render assistance, China must and will turn to others, and she will change her concept of government in the process. If we are not friendly, she may be forced into alliances and treaties which will impose a boycott on America and the western democracies."[72] Not only did humanitarian assistance have the potential to strengthen an international relationship, but the lack thereof could destroy it.

UCR's statement also made clear references to Republican politician Wendell Willkie's "one world" vision, as described in his 1943 book of the same title. After traversing the world by plane in a forty-nine-day trip to four continents, Willkie announced: "There are no distant points in the world any longer. I learned by this trip that the myriad millions of human beings of the Far East are as close to us as Los Angeles is to New York by the fastest trains. I cannot escape the conviction that in the future what concerns them must concern us . . . our thinking in the future must be worldwide."[73] Such right-leaning internationalists connected U.S. interests to global engagement in a way that countered isolationist and noninterventionist elements of Republican politics. As UCR sought to promote Willkie's global vision, it spoke of its work as unique in connecting forces of popular and state initiative. While emphasizing its connection to the recognized government of China, UCR simultaneously portrayed its aid as going beyond the level of the state to connect people to people—an implicit advantage to private work. Education became central to this international popular network, with support of higher education having become increasingly prominent in UCR projects over the course of the 1940s. By 1949, UCR claimed to be supporting 70 percent of China's private universities.[74]

This emphasis on developing an educated elite that might lead China into the future extended into UCR's medical programs, although carried with it its own controversy. Within the ABMAC, debates existed over the extent to which an American model of elite medical education, with its emphasis on research and specialization, should be imported to China. Even those coming out of training in this model through the Peking Union Medical College did not necessarily think it was the best method for China. When the discussion reached UCR, parallels began to appear between the export of both political and medical systems from the U.S. to China. As noted in a 1946 meeting:

> Dr. McConaughy pointed out that their government, although democratic, might not necessarily be the American brand of democracy, and we have no right to impose our type of democracy on the people of China. The American medical profession has a great tendency to impose its form of medicine on China. Dr. McConaughy thinks that China's medical problems are so stupendous that state medicine is the only solution. The American doctors want to train specialists, etc. but Dr. McConaughy is not sure that that would be the best thing for China.[75]

Here, the question of medical infrastructure became intimately linked to political values, demonstrated both by the terms of the debate and the fluidity with which political values were applied to diverse activities, including those of medicine.

Conclusions

This chapter explores the political dimensions and controversies of private U.S. aid to Spain and China as the AMBASD, ABMAC, and CAC began to disintegrate. But it is important to simultaneously recognize that politics were always a part of the foundation of these groups—and, indeed, of the broader history of humanitarian work. What is noteworthy about the controversies highlighted in this chapter is what they reveal about the power claimed by and attributed to private citizens—whether constructive or subversive—as actors in the field of international relations. Hoping to stimulate international action in both private and state spheres, individuals strove to become unofficial diplomats mediating U.S. interactions with the world. Regardless of whether or not they achieved their political aims, the controversy surrounding the activities of individuals involved in the AMBASD, ABMAC, and CAC suggests that both state and private institutions also recognized the potential role of private citizens as intermediaries in international relations. And yet, the changes wrought in the landscape of aid during World War II meant that the space for the individual voluntary impulse was no longer the same.

Conclusions

Although the wars ended in Spain and China, the activism of those involved in the AMBASD and ABMAC did not disappear. While the AMBASD had dissolved, its medical volunteers joined forces with the Veterans of the Abraham Lincoln Brigade (VALB). Remnants of UCR merged with the ABMAC, which followed the exiled Nationalist government to Taiwan. As the Chinese Communists consolidated their power and closed the country to foreign influence, the CAC faded into obscurity. Many of those involved in these campaigns of medical relief found themselves embroiled in heated political debates at home in the U.S. as the ideological battles of the Cold War began to take off in the 1940s. As the decades passed, the fights of many of these activists continued. A number of AMBASD volunteers continued to speak out against Francisco Franco's rule of Spain up until his death in 1975, while members of the ABMAC have continued to support the development of healthcare systems and medical education in Taiwan up until the present day.

Looking beyond World War II, other echoes in private aid may be discovered in other organizations and other campaigns of medical activism. And yet, while each shared something in the seed of individual activism that motivated such efforts, each also reflected differences in the circumstances in which they arose. Nevertheless, the medical activists of the late 1930s set precedents that would resonate with later waves of political activism in the 1960s and 1970s.

The Nicaragua Ambulance Campaign

As the heated debates of the McCarthy period passed, the VALB experienced a renewal in the increasingly liberal climate of the 1960s. Nevertheless, their protests against Franco's Spain had essentially no effect on American foreign policy and rarely even made the mainstream media.[1] For many of the AMBASD's volunteers, Spain became just one chapter in a life of political activism. Like American veterans of the International Brigades, many

AMBASD volunteers found that "political activity had become a matter of habit" and "the surest measure of personal fulfilment and the value of a life's work."[2] During the 1960s, Barsky was involved in providing emergency medical services to civil rights and peace movement workers in the South through the Medical Committee for Human Rights. Martin, who moved to the Pribilof Islands of Alaska in the 1940s, became an activist for Alaska Native rights.[3] After moving to Florida, nurse Rose Wachsman Sorkin played an active role in the Women's International League for Peace and Freedom.[4] In Mexico, nurse Lini De Vries became an advocate for native Mexicans and traveled through rural communities teaching public health.[5]

In the 1980s, the AMBASD inspired the VALB to undertake a fundraising project to send ambulances to Nicaragua. The campaign began with a full-page advertisement in the *New York Times*, drawing parallels between Nicaragua and Spain, while citing veterans' own experiences: "We, the veterans of the Abraham Lincoln Brigade, know that if Hitler, Mussolini, and Franco were alive today, they would support the 'Contras.' To our regret and horror, these forces get most of their support from the CIA. As the first Americans to fight against the Fascist Axis in Spain, we were beneficiaries of medical aid from the people of the U.S.A. Today, we ask for your support in donating a much needed, fully equipped ambulance to the people of Nicaragua."[6] The advertisement raised $100,000 and five ambulances were soon en route to Nicaragua.[7] Meanwhile, three Seattle veterans initiated their own campaign, Northwest to Nicaragua, with the support of other local and regional groups.[8] Through advertisements, letter-writing campaigns, and fundraising events screening *The Good Fight*, Northwest to Nicaragua eventually raised sufficient funds to send three equipped ambulances.

Like the AMBASD, the Nicaragua ambulance campaigns fused political and humanitarian dimensions. As expressed simply in one fundraising letter written from "a medical doctor all too familiar with pain and suffering" to a "fellow human," the objective of the ambulance campaign was described as "humanitarian rather than political or ideological."[9] At the same time, the letter also acknowledged the organization's political interests in describing the situation in Nicaragua, the political complexities, and relevant American foreign policy. The ability to use these varied factors as a fundraising tool was consciously recognized by Northwest to Nicaragua. As noted in a set of directions for fundraisers: "For more sceptical people: Emphasize the humanitarian aspects. Talk about saving lives . . . for enthusiastic people: It's a tangible step to offset official and covert warmongering."[10] The ambulance campaign sought to turn its combined political and humanitarian dimensions into its strength.

AMBASD Political Failures

Just as its later twentieth-century descendant in Nicaragua had done, the AMBASD straddled the contrasting spheres of political campaigning and apolitical humanitarian ideals. The organization's very title reflected this divide in the neutral and official-sounding language of the "American Medical Bureau" followed by the political designation of its purpose "to Aid Spanish Democracy." While the combination of these characteristics may seem contradictory to our understanding of neutral humanitarianism—which the AMBASD referenced in citing its humanitarian focus as distinctly apolitical—both dimensions were crucial parts of the AMBASD's identity. As has been outlined in this study, the AMBASD achieved quantifiable results as an organization seeking to provide medical care to the victims of war, even if its overall impact was relatively small. And its political nature appeared, in hindsight, to be crucial to this success.

On the other hand, if the AMBASD hoped to make its political campaign more successful by emphasizing the humanitarian idealism of its mission, this approach seems to have been less successful. The aim of the combined Medical Bureau and North American Committee to Aid Spanish Democracy to influence American policy toward Spain and lift the embargo was ultimately unsuccessful. As physician and historian Martin Shapiro observed in his analysis of American and British aid to Republican Spain, while "a successful medical aid campaign to people in a military conflict may save some lives," it was unlikely to "affect substantially the course of the conflict," and those "primarily interested in influencing political or military developments . . . may find tactics other than medical aid campaigns more useful in accomplishing their goals."[11]

Shapiro's conclusion operates from the premise of examining the AMBASD as a political campaign with the secondary function of providing medical care. However, this distinction may not necessarily be so facilely applied. While public discourse with the AMBASD's executive officers and committees may indicate organizational priorities, such language seemed to vary depending on who was being asked and when. Drawing larger conclusions about the nature of the AMBASD becomes even more difficult when one looks to the volunteers, as the operational reality of the AMBASD, for clues. Their motivations, as discussed in Chapter 1, varied widely between individuals. Even examining the motivating factors behind one person's decision reveals a complicated picture that is not easily simplified to a single overarching influence. In this sense, the question of whether the AMBASD was driven more by political or humanitarian idealism begins to appear superficial. Again, one must return to the simple fact that both motives played important roles.

ABMAC Political Failures

Turning attention toward the ABMAC, one finds a similar tension between humanitarian idealism and political aims. In the decades following World War II, this became more defined for the ABMAC. From the 1950s onwards, the ABMAC's papers become interspersed with the materials of an organization known as the Committee of One Million. Spearheaded by Nicholas de Rochefort, a Frenchman who renounced French citizenship in 1954 to become an American citizen, the Committee of One Million was a group established to campaign against the admission of a Communist China to the United Nations.[12] De Rochefort found a strong political ally in Congressman (and ABMAC supporter) Dr. Walter B. Judd. Alongside Governor Charles Edison (former UCR president), Frederick C. McKee, Dr. B.A. Garside (a cofounder of UCR and later ABMAC president), and Marvin Lieben, a coalition formed to petition President Eisenhower directly.[13] The group became a vocal lobby, but appears to have failed in collecting its proclaimed one million signatures.

As a political campaign, the ABMAC can also be read as a story of failure in terms of achieving political aims, despite its more prolonged existence. Following the relocation of ABMAC's foreign offices to Taiwan, ABMAC leadership noted, "Without intention, ABMAC has become a factor in America's present-day dilemma of existence, the struggle against Communism. The responsibility has not been sought but it is fully accepted by ABMAC."[14] In his history of the organization, Watt contrasted the Cold War responses of the ABMAC in dedicating "its efforts exclusively to the R.O.C. on Taiwan and principally to Nationalist government medical agencies" with "agencies such as the China Medical Board or the United Board for Christian Higher Education, which diverted their former China funds to colleges throughout East Asia."[15] In so doing, the ABMAC became "an important symbol of moral and political aid to the Nationalist forces struggling to regroup on Taiwan."[16]

Watt attributes much of this laser-like focus and dedication to Nationalist China to Dr. B.A. Garside's leadership as executive director, a position he took over in 1950. That same year, UCR offices merged with the ABMAC's and Garside himself took over the leadership of the ABMAC.[17]

But how did the ABMAC's commitment to the Nationalists in Taiwan actually play out? Their work initially focused on continuing their support of the Nationalist military medical services, but soon expanded into designing a program for civilian health. Although offered $18,000 a month by President Chiang to implement a comprehensive health program in Taiwan, the ABMAC declined the project as beyond the scope of what it realistically might be able to accomplish. Instead, ABMAC representative in China, Dr. Liu, set up a committee in Taiwan to address some of these issues. This advisory role gave the ABMAC something of a blank slate for developing recommendations for Taiwan's civilian and military health system.

Back in the U.S. of the 1950s, debates among the ABMAC faced the challenge of convincing funders that it was still worth fighting for China. As one skeptic wrote to Garside, "After four hundred years, the Chinese have not been able to show any more improvement than to eventually turn to Communism, I hardly think the nation is worth much to work or die for. To say that China has not had the opportunity to move forward is naively absurd."[18] Another "American first-er," as such skeptics came to be labelled, wrote to UCR of his doubts that donations could be made without "interference by present rulers of China," going on to argue that "people of this country should take care of their own, first."[19] For America's China activists, the Communist takeover in 1949 effectively ended all activities on the Chinese mainland. As described in a UCR memo to the State Department's Advisory Committee on Voluntary Foreign Aid:

> As you know, the domination of the China mainland by the Communists has shut off completely the forwarding of funds from the United States for the support of religious, educational, and humanitarian activities there. At present neither USC [UCR] nor any of its member agencies is sending any funds whatever to the China mainland, nor seeking contributions for work in that area. However, some of our agencies are doing all they can to secure assistance for the Chinese people outside of mainland China who are still carrying on the fight against Communism and are working in friendly cooperation with America.[20]

UCR itself as the renamed United Service to China (USC) was "put in mothballs" on 31 December 1950, but maintained a legal existence after and continued collecting unsolicited contributions (which trickled in at a few thousand dollars a month). Terminating the salaries of its employees, but maintaining its same officers and board of directors, it passed any remaining business in aid on to ABMAC. But despite the efforts of a lobby within the U.S. continuing to support Nationalist China, the Communists remained in power and were reported to only have "intensified their restrictions on American religious and humanitarian activities."[21] The anti-foreign element in Communist power even included the CAC, who had been dedicated to their medical assistance during the war.

The Development of Medical Activism

Historian Cary Nelson has claimed that the AMBASD represented the "founding moment of modern medical activism." While a full consideration of Nelson's claim goes beyond the scope of this study, one can certainly find later echoes of the precedent set by the AMBASD (and the other organizations of this study). Throughout the latter half of the twentieth century, a number of more "activist" medical aid organizations developed, consciously striving to bridge the political and medical divide. Médecins Sans Frontières (MSF), or Doctors Without Borders, became one of the most prominent of these, winning the Nobel Peace Prize in 1999 in recognition of its work.

MSF was founded in 1971 by a group of French doctors and journalists driven by dissatisfaction with the perceived failure of states and existing institutions to respond adequately to the victims of the Nigerian Civil War. One of MSF's most prominent founders was highly aware of the Spanish Civil War's tradition of citizen activism. Born in 1939 to a Jewish father, Bernard Kouchner grew up in the shadow of Jewish persecution in World War II. Inspired by the "anti-fascism" of this generation, Kouchner joined the union of Communist students while in medical school.[22] As the conflict in Biafra escalated, it increasingly became Kouchner's own "Spanish Civil War."[23] The story of MSF's foundation shares notable parallels with the organizations we have examined in this study—an awareness and concern for the victims of violence of a foreign conflict, and a fundamental dissatisfaction with the response being mounted by existing institutions. Like these other organizations, the founders of MSF looked to the Red Cross model and sought to differentiate themselves from it, to "[project] the image of a more engaged and daring version" of humanitarian relief.[24] Where the Red Cross was seen to have failed, as a witness who remained silent to many of the atrocities of the World War II, MSF sought to adopt the opposite, to become a witness who would not remain silent. As described by one academic, MSF was "explicitly founded to mediate crisis in terms of human health."[25]

While the world into which the smaller organizations of this study emerged was vastly different, an examination of MSF with its earlier inspiration of international involvement in the Spanish Civil War reveals striking parallels. Descriptions of early MSF missions as "haphazard in organization, largely symbolic in impact, full of romantic panache, and entirely temporary in duration" evoke the AMBASD's activities in Spain.[26] MSF's focus on engaging the media became another quality shared by both—although the latter's ability to do so was limited by the media technology of the day. Nevertheless, one of the most basic volunteer motivations for working with MSF—the opportunity to "feel like a real doctor" in responding directly to a clear medical need—echoes strongly with some of the AMBASD's own volunteers, as Albert Byrne described Spain as offering him the opportunity to "at last be useful" as a doctor.[27]

The professional capacity of the medical volunteer—a more central figure in the AMBASD's work, in contrast to the efforts of the ABMAC or CAC—also became important to their role as witness. As mentioned earlier, a very conscious part of MSF's mission—and a perhaps less conscious, although nearly as important part of the AMBASD's project in Spain—was to transform the medical volunteer into a witness to crisis while addressing the practical and immediate concerns threatening individual health. This privilege, or burden, of observation came with the additional responsibility of publicizing the problems he or she encountered.[28] Doctors, nurses, and other medical personnel had, of course, long been witnesses to the brutal realities of the battlefield. Their more public persona as medical activists, compared by Redfield to traditions of "virtuous testimony" by the public intellectual and gentleman scientist, was a divergence from the Red Cross tradition and "silence" or confidentiality promised by the Hippocratic Oath.[29] At the same time, the physician as public witness seems a natural role to have promoted. The physician was already a professional imbued with moral respectability, whose skills depended largely on his or her power of observation. The physician was also a technical expert backed by the rigorous demands of scientific inquiry—and the objectivity that required.

By these standards, the idea of medical activism reveals itself as a distinct product and reflection of modernity. Medical activists, whether working from the field of battle or in communities at home, have endeavoured to use both the compellingly noble and selfless argument of humanitarian idealism and the respect and authority accorded to the technical expertise of medical professionals to achieve much broader social change. As summarized by Redfield's analysis of MSF's contemporary role in humanitarian relief, "By integrating medical expertise and public expression, the work of this group illustrates an overtly motivated form of scientific research, finding facts in the name of values, in the pursuit of both technical and ethical ends." Redfield goes on to argue that through these methods, "collective actors" such as MSF have come to play a central role in "defining secular moral truth for an international audience."[30] The idea of humanitarianism as defining "secular moral truth" validates claims about its inherent independence from politics.

However, the extent to which the activists behind MSF, or the AMBASD, or the ABMAC, really tried to transcend political questions remains subject to question. After all, as demonstrated in this study, directly embracing the political dimensions and potential implications of aid not only became central to the identities of these organizations, but also gave some of them an initial advantage. However, where the AMBASD and the ABMAC became close affiliates of foreign militaries, MSF has traditionally maintained a greater degree of independence in the field. Nevertheless, one might begin to wonder just how much has really changed since the nineteenth century use of the term "humanitarian"—initially used to negatively describe a political class, much like today's often derogatory reference to the "bleeding-heart liberal."[31] When organizations such as the AMBASD and the ABMAC used the term "humanitarian" to describe their work, alongside their own equally voiced political orientation, questions naturally arise.

While Redfield forms his theories based specifically on MSF, his conclusions are highly relevant for this history as well. Like those of Redfield's study, many in the AMBASD (and similar groups) were concerned with becoming a "moral avatar" of humanitarian effort—the "responsible human" as defined by Redfield.[32] When AMBASD chairman Walter B. Cannon reflected on the role of medical aid in modern war, he admitted the question of such selective aid as practiced by the AMBASD naturally arose. Cannon, however, also equated moral action with some partisanship in noting that "I and persons associated with me in the Medical Bureau sympathize with the legitimate government in Spain, and though we labor with the professional spirit, we apply our main efforts on the side of that government."[33] Cannon became at once a responsible physician striving to relieve human suffering, a responsible citizen seeking to enforce democratic ideals, and a responsible human trying to act in accordance with his own beliefs. Simplified to these basic forms, there is a great sense of continuity between the organizations of this study and later developments such as MSF.

However, there are limits to the comparisons between MSF and the smaller organizations of this study. With their nationally limited foci, it is difficult to equate all with the more global vision promoted by MSF. Although all share a sense of dissatisfaction with contemporary responses to conflict in their roots, whether from existing institutions or state structures, their relationship to the conflicts themselves varied. In contrast to organizations such as the AMBASD in Spain or ABMAC in China, MSF has not sought out the same sort of alliance with foreign military or governmental structures as these organizations did. This may be largely a product of their relative historical contexts. In the later interwar years, with the failure of new international structures such as the League of Nations to contain conflict, there was a slowly growing political consensus toward the limitations of neutrality and the perceived necessity of responding to aggression with force. In the decades following the World War II, amid the tensions of the Cold War, there was perhaps a greater resistance to engaging directly in conflict in the same way.

What stands out in striking contrast between reading the histories of American medical activist organizations in the 1930s as antecedents to MSF is the role of the state and nation within their framework of internationalism. Whereas MSF's title suggests it sought to work explicitly "without borders," organizations such as the AMBASD, ABMAC, and CAC applied their own dissolution of impermeable borders selectively, focusing on connecting the U.S. with a particular nation.[34] These organizations became a mediation of the more negative connotations of nationalism. As historian Karen Minden once observed in writing a study of Chinese medical elite, "When I surmised that the Chinese alumni were motivated by a fervent nationalism, I was gently corrected with the observation that *ai guo*, love of country, was not to be confused with the negative exclusiveness of national sentiment."[35]

The role of nationalist language in the publicity—and mythologies—of the organizations of this study seems to share much with Gary Gerstle's description of American "civic nationalism" in the age of Roosevelt. During this time, Gerstle suggests, nationalism became increasingly painted as something going beyond the boundaries of race and creed, while simultaneously remaining contained by older, racially bound rhetoric.[36] Indeed, Gerstle offers a valuable reexamination of the twentieth century U.S. in contrasting this

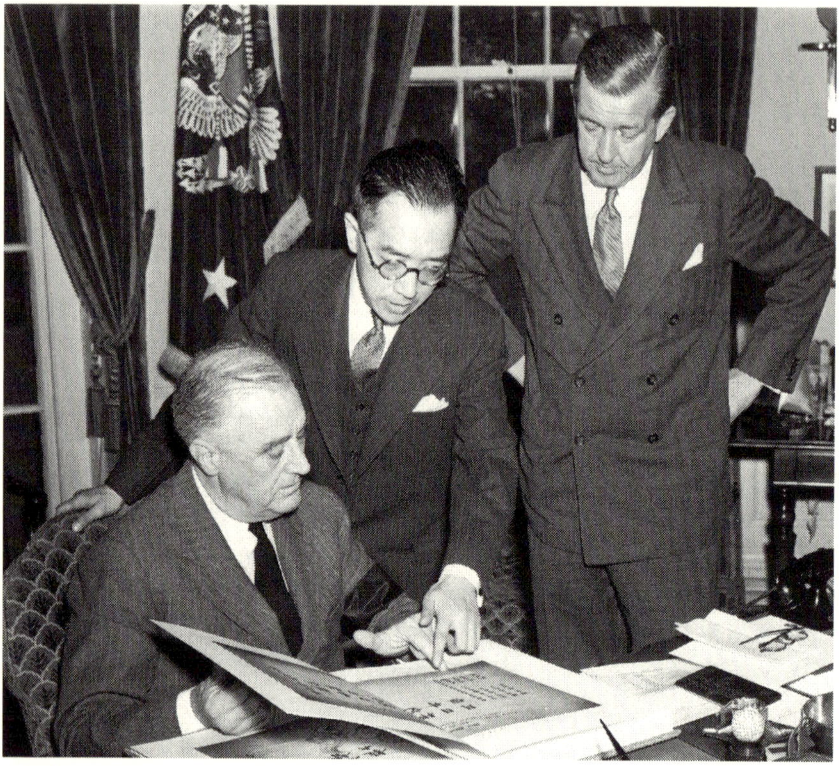

Figure 21. President Roosevelt (left) with Chinese ambassador Hu Shih (middle) and UCR chairman James G. Blaine (right), looking at a Chinese scroll gifted to Roosevelt on the thirtieth anniversary of the Chinese Republic (1942) (USC Records, Mudd Manuscript Library, Princeton University).

"civic nationalism" with "racial nationalism" as two concurrent and competing threads in twentieth-century American history. Using Gerstle's model of American nationalism, the organizations of this study seem to embody an effort of various segments of the American public to expand the American ideal of civic nationalism to an international community. In this, the U.S. still featured prominently—both as a means of translating the importance of these activists' more global vision to American audiences and as an exemplar in their efforts to construct a more global world.

In a broader comparison between MSF and the organizations of this study, UCR stands out slightly from the smaller activist groups we have discussed. In terms of organizational structures, UCR operated on a different scale. Nevertheless, despite its more complex bureaucratic structure and closer affiliation with federal structures, UCR leaders still promoted their work as arising from a grassroots effort. As Edwards once argued to UCR leadership in the U.S., "If [UCR] falls down on its assumed obligations, we are abandoning some of the best social leaders in China, both Chinese and Western, who are working from the grassroots for these ends and have already attained significant results."[37] With the term "grassroots" rooted in politics (describing, according to the *Oxford English Dictionary*, "the rank and file of the electorate or a political party"), it also connotes a segment of the population who might otherwise have limited access or power to enacting social change. The activists of the medical aid organizations of this study were, in this sense, somewhat unique in that many came from a background of greater professional stability and educational investment—or, in other words, from socio-economic strata that tended to have greater access to those dictating formal policy. Because, for many, it was their medical education that gave them that expertise, it became the clearest route for validation of their own political voice when it came to influencing foreign policy.

Even within the category of "medical" relief, however, there were differences of opinion. As Edwards complained of UCR agencies in a letter to Sweet, "They are not ready to consider the needs of China as a whole . . . ABMAC is interested in the national medical education, but is not interested in the general medical program in China . . . the CAC is interested in the general child welfare program in China, but they show a tendency to political prejudice."[38] But while each organization narrowed its vision of its own unique contribution, the claims of the larger impact such contributions would have remained the same. By consciously contributing to the construction of international relationships between the U.S. and other nations, these groups depicted their work as expanding foreign diplomacy into a more popular enterprise going beyond official embassy relations.

As the language of constructing "people-to-people" connections from a grassroots level became more pervasive in private aid efforts, it seems to have trickled into more official state efforts. Writing of its origins in 1947, American Overseas Aid publicity emphasized the personal connections it sought to support in noting that "fundamentally, the anxiety about the world's hungry and homeless is based on a human relationship . . . a relationship between one human being and another human being" and that "between many thousands of human beings, who remember that charity is not an institutional word, but . . . the basis for all our relationships with men and women."[39] Such positive interpersonal dimensions of relief work could feed into U.S. foreign policy interests. As Secretary of State Dean Acheson wrote in a letter to UCR officials in the spring of 1949:

> One of the chief reasons, in my opinion, for the good will and friendly esteem which Americans have always enjoyed in China is the generous, unstinting and sympathetic attitude which private American organizations have inevitably adopted toward the problems which have faced the Chinese . . . It is my hope that during the troubled period through which China is now passing these private American organizations which have contributed so much to the welfare of the Chinese people will not diminish their efforts but will continue insofar as possible the activities which they have so generously supported in the past. I would have no objection to your using or quoting the views which I have expressed in this letter.[40]

The extent to which Acheson's words may be political posturing or sincere may be debated. However, Acheson himself, in his increasingly prominent role in the Truman administration, was one of the key architects behind the development of the Truman Doctrine and, later, the Marshall Plan. Both became defining American policies of the early Cold War, seeking to respond to the threat of Communism through strengthening the economic prosperity of countries (particularly in Europe) believed to be susceptible to Communist control. In both plans, developing positive international relations with the U.S. became a defense against the perceived Communist menace. Using the term "grassroots" as only one example, practitioners of humanitarianism built upon similar language across many types of institutional structures. Regardless of the organization's size, bureaucratic structure, or mission, "grassroots" became a term used to validate humanitarian practice by its own ideals, much like the concept of neutrality.

Between World War I and World War II, the number and types of private organizations expanded exponentially. As cited by Smith, "Fifteen (18.8 percent) of the 80 largest U.S. [private voluntary organizations] in 1980 began in 1918 and 1938."[41] Of these, many were created explicitly for international relief in response to conflict or natural disaster. Between 1919 and 1939, Americans donated more than $8.3 billion to voluntary organizations for work abroad. During this period, the vast majority—70 percent, or $5.8 billion—was directed to recipients through religiously affiliated organizations.[42] Meanwhile, through the Lend-Lease Act, the U.S. spent nearly $50 billion dollars in assistance to over thirty countries.[43] To put these figures in comparison to the effort that followed in World War II, the U.S. government spent $296 billion ($4.014 trillion by today's dollar) on military operations between 1941 and 1945—a figure excluding veterans' benefits, interest on war-related debt, and assistance to allies.[44]

In parallel to the U.S. war effort, the development of aid through the National War Fund offered a more direct method for the U.S. government to encourage and participate in popularizing foreign relief. Displayed geographically, National War Fund projects can be seen paralleling areas of activity in World War II. In 1945 alone the National War Fund appropriated $11,512,452 to UCR.[45] Between 1942 and 1948, UCR and its member agencies directed nearly $50 million in aid to China. Of this, a substantial share (at least $10 million) was dedicated to the medical work of the ABMAC.[46] Prior to National War Fund support, the ABMAC budgeted around $100,000 for their projects abroad and administrative and fundraising activities at home.[47] Between 1944 and 1945, the ABMAC's financial budget had jumped to over $3 million—a 35 percent share of UCR's $9 million total budget.[48] By the last years of the 1940s, however, the ABMAC's income dropped significantly from its wartime levels. In 1948 the ABMAC's income was down to $113,000 and in 1949 it fell to $96,700.[49]

By this time, other institutions of aid were well underway in their development. UNRRA became a major force and "between 1943 and 1947 . . . distributed over $15 billion in resources to war victims and refugees . . . 70% of which was donated by the U.S. government and much of it in food."[50] Although the ARC's first campaign to aid China had failed, by 1943 this had changed. At the end of that year, the ARC reported transmitting $1,190,895.67 of its own funds to China—and disbursing an additional $3,107,091.98 in donations from the U.S. government.[51] In December 1946, having reversed its policy on cash grants, an ARC reported having given $296,081,485.06 in cash grants to the CRC.[52] Considering that the CRC's 1946 campaigns in China raised $689,439,120, the ARC's donations constituted a significant amount.[53]

Meanwhile, money sent to Spain operated on an even smaller scale by its overall financial profile. The highest overall total raised by private groups was, according to historian Richard Traina, approximately $1.8 million.[54] Traina's estimate, however, came from a report reported by the State Department before its completion that its financial figures may be misleading.[55] Beyond this, few newer estimates have been made.

One key difference between the financial realities of aid efforts to Spain and China remains the effect of U.S. entry into the war alongside China. As Sparrow demonstrates in a series of graphs concluding his *Warfare State*, World

War II completely changed U.S. spending priorities and patterns. While U.S. military investment was the most direct recipient of such changes, private aid programs to China, such as those promoted by UCR, found parallel opportunities to tap into these increased resources. Because, ultimately, the money channelled through private aid paled in comparison to overall federal expenditures during this period.

Money and the Myth

UCR itself noted that its real value lay not in the quantities raised, but in its dual "humanitarian and utilitarian purposes," and that "insofar as it does serve these two constructive purposes it is making a contribution to both China and to America far greater than the sums involved."[56] This rationale—in which the high ethical purposes and impacts of humanitarian endeavour rises effortlessly beyond its material reality—is hardly uncommon. In his *Empire of Humanity: A History of Humanitarianism*, Michael Barnett speaks critically, as have others before him, of the self-perpetuated mythology of humanitarianism. According to Barnett, humanitarians often complain about politics and states "encroaching on their turf" with the "world of ethics," even as they "have always defined their turf in political terms."[57] Barnett, like many contemporary historians of humanitarian aid, seeks to correct the suggestion that impartiality and neutrality formed "part of humanitarianism's original DNA." Such may be the myths of humanitarianism, but some of Barnett's critics raise the question of whether Barnett himself creates a new version of this mythology in his historical analysis. As David Rieff writes in review of Barnett: "The less exalting truth, as Barnett surely knows but writes as if he does not know or else does not care, is that people have all sorts of motivations for doing what they do . . . As long as the work they do is valuable, these motivations are of little importance. In the end, Barnett has too much respect for what he believes humanitarianism incarnates as a set of values, an ethics, and too little respect for what humanitarians actually do."[58] It is true, as this study has shown, that the motivations behind the work of self-proclaimed humanitarians are myriad. And there has existed a tendency to allow the language of the ethical and moral high ground humanitarians seek to occupy to overrun the narrative of their history. But, in seeking to redress this imbalance, one can also too easily veer into the baser motives of international interventions. So-called humanitarian work is rarely, if ever, the somehow "pure" and "neutral" endeavour it may promote. Few historians today would argue otherwise, and there has long since been a historical consensus negating the apolitical neutrality of humanitarianism in practice.

However, it is in an examination of the humanitarians themselves that the greatest value of this history resides. Not to draw the sweeping religious conclusions that override motivation, as in Rieff's critique, but to see such actors in their most basic, flawed humanity. In one of his reflections of the Spanish Civil War, James Neugass described an AMBASD nurse giving an extra egg to a Fascist soldier. While one could dissect this episode—and the motivation behind it in any number of ways—it is in the potential impact of this narrative that makes the history of these organizations worth remembering. With the history of the Spanish Civil War still a hotly divisive issue in modern Spain, these stories have the ability to remind people of the moments of human connection in the midst of the inhumanity of war. Even more basically there exists a problem in thinking of the organizations of this study as "humanitarian." Operating from Barnett's contemporary definition of the components of humanitarianism (including humanity, impartiality, neutrality, and independence), it would be a stretch to suggest that the organizations of this study were impartial, neutral, or sought independence from the parties involved. They certainly did, however, maintain a faith in and dedication to humanity. Of course, in certain contexts conflict itself has been labelled "humanitarian" in its purpose and motivation, so one might still question the real difference between such groups and aims.

Final Thoughts

In the end, we return to the argument shared by all the organizations in this study. Despite myriad priorities, the AMBASD, the ABMAC, the CAC, and UCR all justified their existence in their role connecting people to people *and* in supporting a particular foreign interest. In doing so, it was consistently argued, they were building friendships in terms both defined by nationality and superseding it—supporting the relationship between the U.S. and Spain, or the U.S. and China. National identity became implicitly equated with popular identity by American democratic ideals. And such international friendships were almost always framed by the resonance of foreign groups with the democratic traditions of the U.S.—regardless of whether the common connection emphasized was with Communists, Nationalists, or Republicans. Friendships were built, as were new enmities.

American efforts to rally a national effort behind Republican Spain lasted only a few years. Reading into the histories of the foundation of such private efforts, one finds both a critique of U.S. policy and an indifference to it: if the U.S. government and its established agencies for aid would not act, private aid would. Efforts to effect change were therefore directed predominantly at the American people, rather than toward the government itself. In China, the effort lasted longer, fueled by Sino-American cooperation in World War II. Again, organizations such as the ABMAC and CAC illustrate some of the same tension between critique of and indifference toward U.S. foreign policy in turning to private action in their founding. However, changing external circumstances led these groups into closer collaboration with U.S. governmental structures in their pursuit of foreign policy objectives. The people of the ABMAC and the CAC sought to redress this perceived imbalance by becoming proactive in mediating Sino-American relations as individual citizens. The leaders of UCR pursued many of the same goals, but where the ABMAC and CAC turned first to foreign Chinese leadership, UCR prioritized different channels. The conflicts that arose within UCR surrounding these organizations were largely disagreements over those channels of aid. But do any of these details and disagreements mark any real change in diplomatic history? Diplomatic history has always, in part, consisted of the stories of individual interactions between persons. However, as global communication increasingly connected different parts of the world, this study argues that private citizens became more proactive in seeking to mediate such relations themselves.

During this earlier period and in contrast to later organizations such as MSF, value was still connected to national and political identities. The ABMAC wanted to help the Nationalists, to make their vision China's future. The CAC had their own vision, allied with the Chinese Communists. The AMBASD had its own vision for Spain, which was as much a reaction against the perceived threat of Fascism in Europe as it was connected to any particular vision for Spain itself. Ultimately these limitations in their view of internationalism would cause their disintegration. As much as their language described a broad and all-inclusive internationalism, in practice it was still limited by nationality. In later eras, similar responses to foreign conflict would arise—as grassroots responses arising from sympathy for the victims of foreign lands. Some of these would remain, like the organizations discussed in this chapter, tied to nationalism. However, over the course of the twentieth century, the language of international aid increasingly moved away from the "nation" as a unit defining the world, as we can see in the increase of new terms of international relations, from the transnational to the global.[59]

While still relying on the term "international," *A Different Kind of Diplomacy*, edited by Dr. Jack Fisher in 1987, describes the same type of citizen movement. In the forward to this edited collection, Dr. Armand Hammer relates the story of his involvement in mounting a private American response to the Chernobyl disaster in the Soviet Union. As Hammer states, "I am a firm believer in the concept that one individual can, and does make a difference, and that one of the highest rewards available to humans is the opportunity to contribute in however small a way, to the better good of mankind."[60] Hammer had been involved in medical aid to the Soviet Union since the 1920s, first traveling there as a recent medical school graduate waiting to begin an internship. Hammer appears to have been independently wealthy, as he describes mounting a private effort—with his own resources—to supply grain, ambulance, and medical supplies. From these efforts, Hammer reported the Communist government of the U.S.S.R. granted Hammer a number of business concessions that ultimately led him to shift from the practice of medicine to the practice of international business. In the end, Hammer concludes:

> I believe my experiences, only a few of which I have described here, point to the importance of private citizens offering their own kind of help to people of other countries. I would emphasize, however, that I do believe that such assistance while it can be and often is independent of government action and policy, should nevertheless be in accordance with U.S. government policies and beliefs. It can act as a complement to official policy and perhaps serve as a bridge to help bring nations closer together in pursuit of the common goals of peace and a better life for all mankind.[61]

James Sparrow has suggested that understanding the cultural foundations of collective political action has all too often occupied a blind spot for historians and political scientists alike. He argues that rather than restricting analyses to lofty ideologies or the proclamations of pressure groups, a focus on "the interplay between state formation and political culture at the grassroots" makes it possible "to uncover the shared assumptions that ordered both cooperation and conflict within the polity."[62] This study may offer a small contribution into understanding a cultural tradition of humanitarian endeavour—and from that basis, present a glimpse into the tremendously multifactorial nature of American foreign relations in practice. Rather than attempt to reduce either history—that of humanitarian development, or that of American foreign relations—to a dominant theme, this study tries to identify many. Although certain groups held more power than others, change arose not from the control of any one group or individual.

But, perhaps most importantly, tracing private aid efforts in the period of transition marked by World War II confirms the war's role as a major turning point in the balance between private and governmental power. Amid the exigencies of war, would-be critics of U.S. policy generally pursued ways of embracing federal power and seeking to use it to their own advantage, rather than protest or dismantle it.[63] AMBASD attempts to bend U.S. foreign policy toward the cause of Spain inspired those of ABMAC to take a different political tact, while UCR's entrance surpassed both in finding federal allies. While the organizations of this study varied in their challenges and criticism to federal efforts, all remained consistent in establishing a political voice as a symbiotic companion to humanitarian intervention. From the small private efforts of medical activism, state structures and transnational institutions developed during and after World War II fundamentally changed the landscape of U.S. aid. These changes ultimately limited the potential impact of private medical activism under the models developed by groups such as the AMBASD and ABMAC. Medical aid would continue to be pursued as a response to conflict, and with the expansion of the U.S. Department of Defense, continue to play a role in both military strategy and foreign policy. The space for individual citizens to be at the forefront of such efforts would not, however, be the same. But the activism of those involved in private aid to Spain and China still tells an important story of the more complex internationalism of the U.S. in the 1930s and the development of new standards of aid in conflict.

Appendix A

AMBASD Volunteer Profile

Doctors

Nearly thirty physicians and surgeons traveled to Spain on behalf of the AMBASD. All but one were men. Their ages ranged from mid-twenties to mid-fifties. They came from all over the U.S., although a particularly strong contingent (roughly half) came from New York and other major cities of the Northeast. Six were immigrants, four coming from Russia, one from England, and one from Spain. Many were single when they traveled to Spain, although a few were married with families. The vast majority were of Jewish heritage, although only a handful self-identified their religion as such.[1] While many seem to have been involved with or sympathetic to liberal and progressive political causes besides Spain, only three are definitely known to have been members of the Communist Party. At least five attended medical school or completed post-graduate medical training in Europe.

Nurses

By the end of the war, over fifty women (and at least one man) had volunteered in Spain as nurses with the AMBASD. Most were in their twenties, although some were in their mid-thirties, and at least one was forty to fifty years old at the time. Almost all were single—many of them were only a few years out of nurse training. As with the doctors, the nurses came from all over the U.S., with a particularly large percentage coming from New York and the Northeast. At least nine were immigrants, coming mostly from Russia and Eastern Europe. Two of these were Dutch immigrants. One nurse was African American. At least nine identified themselves as Jewish, one as Catholic, and one as Protestant. Several—including some of those mentioned above—described themselves as agnostic or nonpracticing, regardless of their background. While many clearly identified with liberal and progressive politics, only three of those who completed Martin's later questionnaire claim to have been members of the Communist Party.[2]

Other

AMBASD units also included many other types of medically qualified personnel. The dental unit included four dentists and three or four dental assistants. Five laboratory technicians, one x-ray technician, and one pharmacist also worked for the AMBASD in Spain. Both Eugenia Grunsky and Luba Brisker were physical therapists, although the latter was also a trained nurse. The demographics of this somewhat disparate group appear relatively comparable to the doctors and nurses involved. At least two were immigrants—one from Peru and the other from Russia. Though volunteers came from all of the U.S., the largest concentration came from New York. At least two classified their religion as Jewish, and one as Protestant.

Although most volunteers involved in the AMBASD's work in Spain were individuals with professional qualifications—such as doctors, nurses, dentists, and medical assistants or technicians—people without such qualifications were just as integral to AMBASD's program of medical relief. The AMBASD also recruited ambulance drivers and chauffeurs, mechanics and engineers, and administrative staff to support the medical units. Such support staff traveled with almost every unit to sail to Spain. Mildred Rackley, an acquaintance of Barsky's and a fluent Spanish speaker, accompanied the first group as a hospital administrator and translator. For others, the role of support staff provided an opportunity for spouses to accompany loved ones to Spain—although the AMBASD generally tried to avoid sending married couples to Spain together because of the personal complications this might cause in the field.[3] Helene Weissman, who worked in the AMBASD's New York office, was asked to take her administrative skills to Spain, where she joined her husband, physician Oscar Weissman.[4] Alba Novac worked as a cook and general assistant. Her husband, too, was already in Spain, although as a volunteer in the International Brigades.[5] Ambulance driver Evelyn Rahman eventually joined her husband in Spain as well. Although both of the Rahmans had applied to become ambulance drivers with the First Unit, only Carl had been accepted. Besides the AMBASD's unwritten policy of trying to avoid sending husband and wife together, Evelyn had to battle against a male leadership that initially questioned her ability to be a driver—a task generally assigned to men.[6] She nevertheless became a valuable addition and popular figure both in Spain and in AMBASD promotional literature at home.

Ambulance Drivers

The AMBASD sent over twenty drivers to Spain as recruits from the U.S., while a number of others joined AMBASD services once there. Driving an ambulance proved a relatively popular way for injured members of the International Brigades to continue to stay involved in some aspect of the war effort while they recovered. The ambulance driver had achieved a new status since World War I. American writers such as Ernest Hemingway and John Dos Passos—both of whom had driven ambulances in World War I and actively spoke out on behalf of the Republic during the Spanish Civil War—helped popularize the figure of ambulance driver as hero. Compared to other groups of volunteers with the AMBASD, relatively little is known about the ambulance drivers as a whole. At least five were immigrants from Spain, with clear personal or familial ties supporting their decision to volunteer. At least one was an African American. James Neugass's recently published memoir, *War Is Beautiful*, offers the most extensive portrait to date of an AMBASD ambulance driver, in addition to offering a glimpse into the personal details of a handful of others. Neugass himself, like a number of other AMBASD volunteers, was Jewish and spent time in New York (in addition to traveling extensively in Europe), although was originally from New Orleans.[7]

Following the examples set by Hemingway, Dos Passos and others, a number of drivers also had artistic or literary interests. James Neugass, already discussed, offers a prime example of this. Although his first published novel came after the war, his work had been published in a number of journals of poetry before. Judson Briggs was already an established artist in the United States. His activism in favor of Republican Spain not only drove him to volunteer with the AMBASD as a driver, but also led to an artistic exhibition held in his honor in Paris in April 1938.[8] Showcasing seventeen of Briggs's own paintings, alongside a study of Picasso's famous *Guernica*, this exhibition was another important method of publicizing the work of organizations such as the AMBASD and CSI while promoting the cause of the Spanish Republic. Other drivers doubled as correspondents, using their experiences working in the midst of the conflict as a springboard for writing their own commentary on the conflict. Whatever their other interests may have been, the ambulance drivers of the AMBASD did more than just drive vehicles—they served as general "handymen" for the medical services throughout Spain. As lab technician Dorothy Fontaine fondly recalled, "My greatest admiration . . . was for the Ambulance drivers. They were ingenious, imaginative and coped with their problems in an extremely efficient way."[9]

Appendix B

Map of the AMBASD in Spain

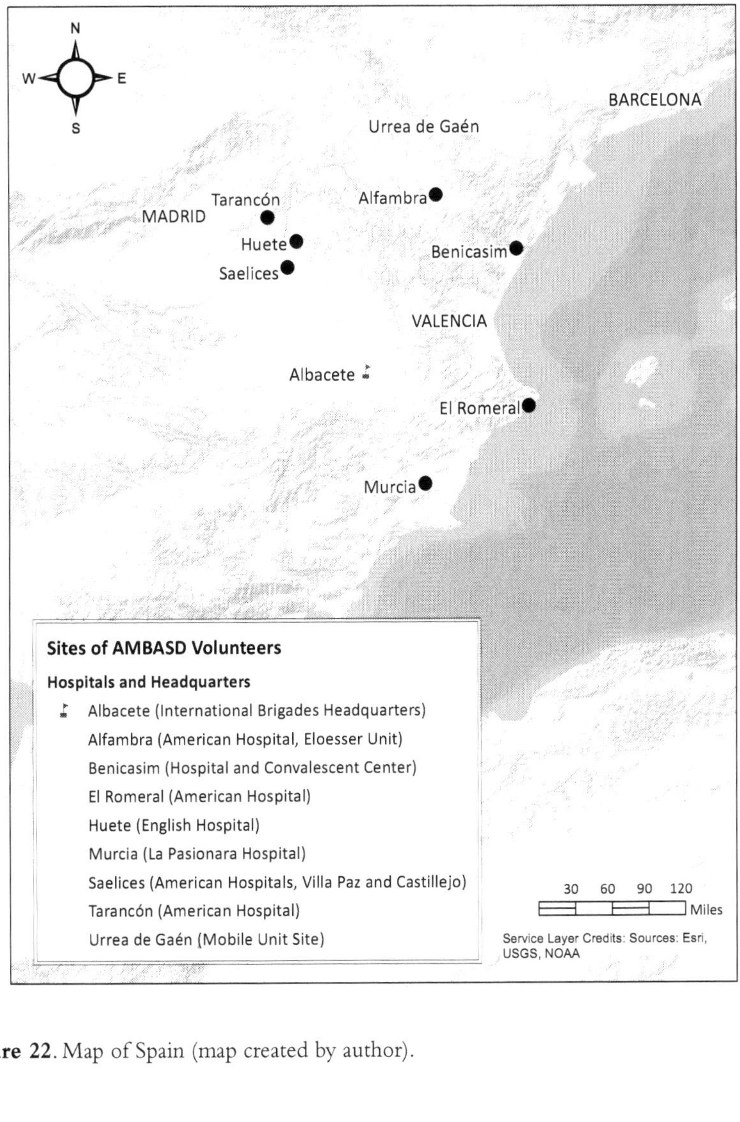

Figure 22. Map of Spain (map created by author).

Notes

An Introduction

1. Ian R. Tyrrell, *Transnational Nation: United States History in Global Perspective since 1789* (Basingstoke, UK: Palgrave Macmillan, 2007).

2. Mabel Boardman, "Mabel T. Boardman of the American Red Cross on Medical Aid in Modern War," *Journal of the Association of Medical Students* (1938): 164–165.

3. Brian Balogh, *A Government Out of Sight: The Mystery of National Authority in Nineteenth Century America* (Cambridge: Cambridge University Press, 2009).

4. Walter B. Cannon, "Walter B. Cannon on Medical Aid in Modern War," *Journal of the Association of Medical Students* (1938)

5. Julia Irwin, "Humanitarian Occupations: Foreign Relief and Assistance in the Formation of American International Identities, 1898–1928" (unpublished PhD diss., Yale University, 2009); Saul Benison, Clifford A. Barger, and Elin L. Wolfe, "Walter B. Cannon and the Mystery of Shock: Study of Anglo-American Cooperation in World War I," *Medical History* 35 (1991): 221.

6. Cannon, "Walter B. Cannon on Medical Aid in Modern War."

7. Ibid.

8. Ibid.

9. Exceptions may be found in Tom Buchanan's recent work and a handful of biographical studies of medical volunteers who traveled first to Spain and then to China. Tom Buchanan, "'Shanghai-Madrid Axis'? Comparing British Responses to the Conflicts in Spain and China, 1936–1949," *Contemporary European History* 21 (2012): 533–552; Tom Buchanan, *East Wind: China and the British Left, 1925–1976* (Oxford: Oxford University Press, 2012).

10. Relatively few Americans volunteered both in Spain and China, although some U.S. organizations contributed to aiding both conflicts. A handful of medical personnel from other countries, however, did travel to China following their time in Spain. Angela Jackson, *For Us It Was Heaven: The Passion, Grief & Fortitude of Patience Darton—From the Spanish Civil War to Mao's China* (Sussex: Sussex Academic Press, 2012); G.E. Sichon, "Mémoires Et Témoignages, Les Médicins Des Deux Guerres: Espagne 1936–1939, Chine 1939–1945," *Matériaux pour l'histoire de notre temps* 19 (1990): 57–64.

11. Dennis Merrill and Thomas G. Paterson, ed., *Major Problems in American Foreign Relations: Documents and Essays*, 7th ed. 2 vols. (Boston: Wadsworth Cengage Learning, 2010), II. The most recent edition, for example, jumps from "Chapter 3:

The International History of the Twenties" to "Chapter 4: U.S. Entry into World War II." A similar gap is found in: Thomas Bender, *A Nation among Nations: America's Place in World History* (New York: Hill & Wang, 2006).

12. Akira Iriye, *Global Community: The Role of International Organizations in the Making of the Contemporary World* (Berkeley: University of California Press, 2002), 1. See also: Iriye, "The Internationalization of History," *American Historical Review* 94 (1989): 1–10; Iriye, "The Role of International Organizations," in *The Global History Reader*, ed. Bruce Mazlish and Akira Iriye (New York: Routledge, 2005); Iriye, *Cultural Internationalism and World Order* (Baltimore: Johns Hopkins University Press, 1997).

13. Tyrrell, *Woman's World, Woman's Empire: The Woman's Christian Temperance Union in International Perspective, 1880–1930* (Chapel Hill: University of North Carolina Press, 1991); Tyrrell, *Reforming the World: The Creation of America's Moral Empire* (Princeton: Princeton University Press, 2010); Tyrrell, *Transnational Nation: United States History in Global Perspective Since 1789.*

14. Y.S. Wang and T.O. Cheng, "Leo Eloesser: An American Cardiothoracic Surgeon in China," *Annals of Thoracic Surgery* 71 (2001): 1387–1388.

15. Bertrand Taithe, "The Red Cross Flag in the Franco-Prussian War: Civilians, Humanitarians, and War in the 'Modern Age,'" in *War, Medicine and Modernity*, ed. Roger Cooter, Mark Harrison, and Steve Sturdy (Stroud: Sutton Publishing, 1998).

16. Emily S. Rosenberg, "Missions to the World: Philanthropy Abroad," in *Charity, Philanthropy, and Civility in American History*, ed. Lawrence J. Friedman and Mark D. McGarvie (Cambridge: Cambridge University Press, 2003), 251.

17. Beginning with President Truman's Marshall Plan, humanitarian aid became an increasingly integral tool to policymakers seeking to push an alternative political system to the Communist world of the Soviet Union in the years following World War II.

18. Marta Rey García, *Stars for Spain: La Guerra Civil Española en los Estados Unidos* (Madrid: Ediciós de Castro, 1995)

19. Davies's history of the FAU during World War II offers a useful account of the China Convoy's work. A. Tegla Davies, *Friends Ambulance Unit: The Story of the F.A.U. in the Second World War 1939–1946* (London: George Allen and Unwin Limited, 1947).

20. Margaret Stanley, the first American nurse to join the China Convoy, later wrote of her experiences after revisiting the country in 1972 with the AFSC. Margaret Stanley, "China: Then and Now," *American Journal of Nursing* 72 (1972): 2213–2218; Stanley, "Two Experiences of an American Public Health Nurse in China a Quarter of a Century Apart," *American Journal of Public Health* 63 (1973): 111–116. British volunteer John E. Simpson later published a collection of letters to his future wife, which provide a firsthand account of the China Convoy's activities. John E. Simpson, *Letters from China: Quaker Relief Work in Bandit Country, 1944–1946* (Cambridge: Ross-Evans, 2001).

21. Sydney D. Bailey, "Review of Quaker Relief: An Account of the Relief Work of the Society of Friends," *International Affairs* 29 (1953): 270.

22. Davies, *Friends Ambulance Unit*, 288.

23. Historian Lisa McGirr has established a valuable model for this. See: Lisa McGirr, "The Interwar Years," in *American History Now*, ed. Eric Foner and Lisa McGirr, Critical Perspectives on the Past (Philadelphia: Temple University Press, 2011).

24. Robert Dallek, *Franklin D. Roosevelt and American Foreign Policy, 1932–1945* (Oxford: Oxford University Press, 1995).

25. Warren I. Cohen, *Empire without Tears: America's Foreign Relations, 1921–1933* (New York: Alfred A. Knopf, 1987); Iriye, "Internationalization of History"; Iriye, *Cultural Internationalism and World Order.*

26. Cohen, *Empire without Tears*, 138.

27. Dallek, *Franklin D. Roosevelt and American Foreign Policy*, 102. The Nye Committee conducted hearings between September 1934 and February 1936, investigating American involvement in World War I. The committee found questionable ties between U.S. foreign policy and the financial interests of the munitions industry, concluding that corporate interests had held too much sway in deciding American state policy.

28. Eric R. Smith, *American Relief Aid and the Spanish Civil War* (Columbia: University of Missouri Press, 2013).

29. Dallek, *Franklin D. Roosevelt and American Foreign Policy*, 102.

30. For more on the volunteers of the Abraham Lincoln Brigade; see: Peter N. Carroll, *The Odyssey of the Abraham Lincoln Brigade: Americans in the Spanish Civil War* (Palo Alto, CA: Stanford University Press, 1994); Allen Guttman, *The Wound in the Heart: America and the Spanish Civil War* (New York: Free Press, 1962). For more on the International Brigades as a whole; see: Antonio R. Celada, Daniel Pastor García and Rosa M. López Alonso, ed., *Las Brigadas Internacionales: 70 Años De Memoria Histórica* (Salamanca: Amarú Ediciones, 2007). For Britain's contributions to the International Brigades; see: Tom Buchanan, *Britain and the Spanish Civil War* (Cambridge: Cambridge University Press, 1997).

31. Chennault served as a consult to the Chinese air force since the outbreak of the war in 1937, enlisting a number of American pilots to join Chinese forces in their fight against the Japanese in 1939. Yuwu Song, ed., *Encyclopedia of Chinese-American Relations* (Jefferson, NC: McFarland & Co., 2006).

32. Carl Molesworth, *Sharks over China: The 23rd Fighter Group in World War II* (Washington D.C.: Brassey's, 1994).

33. Merle Eugene Curti, *American Philanthropy Abroad* (New Brunswick, NJ: Rutgers University Press, 1963), 22.

34. Red Ross, "Black Americans and Italo-Ethiopian Relief 1935–1936", in *Race and U.S. Foreign Policy from the Colonial Period to the Present,* ed. Michael Krenn (London: Routledge, 1998), 170.

35. Danny Duncan Collum, ed., *African Americans in the Spanish Civil War: "This Ain't Ethiopia, But It'll Do"* (New York: G.K. Hall, 1992), 19–20.

36. Bertrand M. Patenaude, *The Big Show in Bololand: The American Relief Expedition to Soviet Russia in the Famine of 1921* (Palo Alto: Stanford University Press, 2002).

37. Julia Irwin's *Making the World Safe* offers the most up-to-date account of the initial development of the ARC. Dulles's somewhat dated account offers a broader chronological overview of ARC history, contrasted with the critical account offered by Shealy. Julia Irwin, *Making the World Safe: The American Red Cross and a Nation's Humanitarian Awakening* (Oxford: Oxford University Press, 2013); Foster Rhea Dulles, *The American Red Cross: A History* (Westport, CT: Greenwood Press, 1950); Gwendolyn C. Shealy, *A Critical History of the American Red Cross, 1882–1945: The End of Noble Humanitarianism* (Lewiston, NY: Edwin Mellen Press, 2003). Several doctoral dissertations have also contributed, including: Thomas H. Reynolds, "American Red Cross Disaster Services, 1930–1947" (unpublished Ph.D. diss., New York: Columbia University, 1954); Marian Moser Jones, "Confronting Calamity: The American Red Cross and the Politics of Disaster Relief, 1881–1939" (unpublished PhD diss., Columbia University, 2008).

38. Paul Weindling, ed., *International Health Organisations and Movements, 1918–1939* (Cambridge: Cambridge University Press, 1995).

39. David C. Hammack, "Failure and Resilience: Pushing the Limits in Depression and Wartime," in *Charity, Philanthropy, and Civility in American History*, ed. Lawrence J. Friedman and Mark D. McGarvie (Cambridge: Cambridge University Press, 2003).

40. Rosenberg, "Missions to the World: Philanthropy Abroad"; Tyrrell, *Reforming the World: The Creation of America's Moral Empire*; Curti, *American Philanthropy Abroad*.

41. See: Tommy G. Thompson, "The Cure for Tyranny," *Boston Globe*, 24 October 2005; Major Jay B. Baker, "Medical Diplomacy in Full-Spectrum Operations," *Military Review*, Sept–Oct 2007; Donald F. Thompson, "The Role of Medical Diplomacy in Stabilizing Afghanistan," *Defense Horizons*, No. 63, May 2008; David S. Broder, "Diplomacy That Heals," *Washington Post*, 15 January 2009.

42. Bruno Cabanes, *The Great War and the Origins of Humanitarianism, 1918–1924* (Cambridge: Cambridge University Press, 2014), 5–10.

43. Michelle Tusan, *Smyrna's Ashes: Humanitarianism, Genocide, and the Birth of the Middle East* (Berkeley: University of California Press, 2012); Keith David Watenpaugh, *Bread from Stones: The Middle East and the Making of Modern Humanitarianism* (Oakland: University of California Press, 2015).

44. Tusan, *Smyrna's Ashes*, 7.

45. Robert H. Bremner, *American Philanthropy* (Chicago: University of Chicago Press, 1988); James T. Sparrow, *Warfare State: World War II Americans and the Age of Big Government* (New York: Oxford University Press, 2011); Olivier Zunz, *Philanthropy in America: A History* (Princeton: Princeton University Press, 2011).

46. Sparrow, *Warfare State*, 7.

47. Zunz, *Philanthropy in America*.

48. Michael Barnett, *Empire of Humanity: A History of Humanitarianism* (Ithaca: Cornell University Press, 2011); Michael Barnett and Thomas George Weiss, *Humanitarianism Contested: Where Angels Fear to Tread* (Milton Park, England: Routledge, 2011); Michael Barnett and Thomas George Weiss, ed., *Humanitarianism in Question: Politics, Power, Ethics* (Ithaca: Cornell University Press, 2008).

49. In comparison to their American colleagues, British historians have directed greater attention to the "Aid Spain" movement in Britain. For an overview of the British aid movement; see: Jim Fyrth, *The Signal Was Spain: The Spanish Aid Movement in Britain, 1936–1939* (London: Lawrence & Wishart, 1986). Angela Jackson's work offers another interesting perspective on aid workers in Spain; see: *British Women and the Spanish Civil War* (London: Routledge, 2002); *Beyond the Battlefield: Testimony, Memory, and Remembrance of a Cave Hospital* (Pontypool: Warren & Pell Publishing, 2005); and *At the Margins of Mayhem* (Pontypool: Warren & Pell Publishing, 2008). Tom Buchanan offers some critical alternatives to Fyrth and Jackson's interpretation of the politics of the British aid movement, found in his reviews of their work. See: "Britain's Popular Front?: Aid Spain and the British Labour Movement," *History Workshop Journal* 31/1 (1991); and "Review of Angela Jackson, British Women and the Spanish Civil War," H-Albion, *H-Net Reviews* (September 2003). and in selected chapters of his books, *Britain and the Spanish Civil War* and *The Impact of the Spanish Civil War on Britain: War, Loss and Memory* (Brighton: Sussex Academic Press 2007).

50. Smith, *American Relief Aid.*

51. Julia Newman (dir.), "Into the Fire: American Women in the Spanish Civil War" (First Run Features, 2002); Frances Patai, "Heroines of the Good Fight: Testimonies of U.S. Volunteer Nurses in the Spanish Civil War, 1936–1939," *Nursing History Review*, 3 (1995): 79–104.

52. Rey García, *Stars for Spain.*

53. Gabriel Jackson, *The Spanish Republic and the Civil War, 1931–1939* (Princeton: Princeton University Press, 1965), 430–450.

54. José Ramón Navarro Carballo, *La Sanidad en las Brigadas Internacionales* (Madrid, 1989); José M. Massons, *Historia de la Sanidad Militar Española* (Barcelona: Ediciones Pomares-Corredor, 1994); Manuel Requena and Rosa Mª Sepúlveda, eds., *La Sanidad en las Brigadas Internacionales* (Cuenca, 2006); Francisco Guerra, *La Medicina en el Exilio Republicano* (Madrid: Servicio de Publicaciones del Estado Mayor del Ejercito, 2003); Celada, García, and López Alonso, *Las Brigadas Internacionales.*

55. Nicolas Coni, *Medicine and Warfare: Spain, 1936–1939* (New York, 2008).

56. For instance, at the "English Hospital" in Huete, American Mildred Rackley played an important role as administrator and translator—and American nurse Thelma Erickson also visited. Manuel Olarte Madero, *Las Brigadas Internacionales: El "Hospital Inglés De Huete"* (Cuenca: Servicio de Publicaciones del Estado Mayor del Ejercito, 2010); Linda Palfreeman, *¡Salud! British Volunters in the Republican Medical Service During the Spanish Civil War, 1936–1939* (Eastbourne: Sussex Academic Press, 2012).

57. Carroll, *Odyssey of the Abraham Lincoln Brigade.*

58. Carroll mentions three doctors (Edward Barsky, Irving Busch, and the Canadian Norman Bethune), one nurse (Fredericka Martin), one ambulance driver (Milt Felsen), and one pharmacist (Harry Wilkes).

59. The seven other agencies involved in UCR's campaign included the China Emergency Relief Committee, Inc., the China Aid Council; the American Committee for Chinese War Orphans, Inc.; Indusco, Inc.; the Associated Boards for Christian Colleges in China; the Church Committee for China Relief; and China Famine Relief.

60. Mudd Manuscript Library, Princeton University, United Service to China Records, Box 4, Folder 7: "Past Achievements and Present Program."

61. "$5,000,000 Sought for China Relief," *New York Times*, 3 March 1941.

62. Patricia Neils, China Images in the Life and Times of Henry Luce (Savage, MD: Rowman & Littlefield Publishers, Inc., 1990). Barbara W. Tuchman, *Stilwell and the American Experience in China, 1911–1945* (New York: Macmillan Company, 1971); James C. Thomson Jr., *While China Faced West: American Reformers in Nationalist China, 1928–1937* (Cambridge, MA: Harvard University Press, 1969); Michael Schaller, *The U.S. Crusade in China, 1938–1945* (New York: Columbia University Press, 1979); Michael Schaller, *The United States and China: Into the Twenty-First Century* (New York: Oxford University Press, 2002); Warren I. Cohen, *America's Response to China: An Interpretive History of Sino-American Relations* (New York: John Wiley & Sons, Inc., 1971); Mary Brown Bullock, *An American Transplant: The Rockefeller Foundation and Peking Union Medical College* (Berkeley: University of California Press, 1980).

63. "China Honors Seven Here," *New York Times*, 28 October 1942.

64. An exception may be found in the efforts of independent historian and former ABMAC president John R. Watt. John R. Watt, *A Friend in Deed: ABMAC and the Republic of China, 1937–1987* (New York: ABMAC Foundation, 1992); Watt, ed., *Health Care and National Development in Taiwan, 1950–2000*, ed. John R. Watt (New York: ABMAC Foundation, 2008).

65. Bullock, *An American Transplant.*

66. Alan Brinkley, *The Publisher: Henry Luce and His American Century* (New York: Alfred A. Knopf, 2010); Jespersen, *American Images of China;* Neils, *China Images in the Life and Times of Henry Luce*; Karen J. Leong, *The China Mystique: Pearl S. Buck, Anna May Wong, Mayling Soong, and the Transformation of American Orientalism* (Berkeley: University of California Press, 2005); Vanessa Künnemann, "'Following with Bleeding Footsteps?' American Missions in China and the (Gendered) Critique of Pearl S. Buck," in Trans-Pacific Interactions: The United States and China, 1880–1950, ed. Vanessa Künnemann and Ruth Mayer (New York: Palgrave Macmillan, 2009).

67. Kenneth E. Shewmaker, *Americans and Chinese Communists, 1927–1945: A Persuading Encounter* (Ithaca: Cornell University Press, 1971), 270.

68. One example of the latter is Canadian physician and medical missionary Dr. Richard Brown. Shewmaker, *Americans and Chinese Communists*, 92.

69. Ruth V. Hemenway, *Ruth V. Hemenway, M.D.: A Memoir of Revolutionary China, 1924–1941* (Amherst: University of Massachusetts Press, 1977).

70. Bethune has received significant attention as an outstanding figure for his work in both Spain and China. Dying from sepsis during his service in China, he has since been promoted to the status of hero in China. For biographical accounts; see: Ted Allan and Sydney Gordon, *The Scalpel, the Sword: The Story of Dr. Norman Bethune* (New York: Monthly Review Press, 1973); Roderick Stewart and Sharon Stewart, *Phoenix: The Life of Norman Bethune* (Montreal: McGill-Queens University Press, 2012).

71. Sidney Shapiro, *Ma Haide: The Saga of American Doctor George Hatem in China* (Beijing: Foreign Languages Press, 2004).

72. Franklin Delano Roosevelt, "Radio Address on the National War Fund," 5 Oct online at http://www.presidency.ucsb.edu/ws/index.php?pid=16322; Rosenberg, "Missions to the World: Philanthropy Abroad," 256; Hyde Park, Franklin D. Roosevelt Library, Franklin D. Roosevelt, Papers as President: Official File, Box 1, Folder 5229: Letter, Prescott W. Bush to General Watson, 23 March 1943.

73. Rosenberg, "Missions to the World: Philanthropy Abroad"; Emily S. Rosenberg, *Spreading the American Dream: American Economic and Cultural Expansion, 1890–1945* (New York: Hill & Wang, 1982); Brenda Gayle Plummer, "The Changing Face of Diplomatic History: A Literature Review," *History Teacher* 38 (2005): 385–400.

74. Smith also noted that many black nationalist leaders supporting aid to Ethiopia complained vocally about these connections, although others, such as Langston Hughes, became intimately involved in the causes of both Ethiopia and Spain. Smith, *American Relief Aid and the Spanish Civil War.*

One Americans Respond: The Development of Private Aid

1. Buchanan, "'Shanghai-Madrid Axis'? Comparing British Responses to the Conflicts in Spain and China, 1936–1949."

2. All four of these cities were targets of major bombing raids, causing significant civilian deaths, and earning substantial press coverage as a result. Buchanan links these in his comparative study, "Shanghai-Madrid Axis," particularly in the peak of their shared press coverage in 1937. While this author has not done an exhaustive search of U.S. periodical coverage of both wars, a number of articles comparing atrocities in both can be found—with the greatest focus on civilian threats by aerial bombardment first appearing in 1937. Otto D. Tolischus, "Berlin Darkened in Vast War Test," *New York Times*, 21 September 1937; Hanson W. Baldwin, "The Fear of Flying Death Darkens: Europe's Skies," *New York Times*, 26 September 1937; Hanson W. Baldwin, "Spain and China Suffer in Wars that Drag On," *New York Times*, 9 October 1938; "War Safety Zones Urged," *New York Times*, 16 September 1939.

3. Edward Barsky, "The Surgeon Goes to War," Box 5, Folders 4–21, Edward Barsky Papers, Tamiment Library, New York University, New York. [Hereafter: Barsky, "The Surgeon."]

4. Smith, *American Relief Aid and the Spanish Civil War.*

5. There were a number of exceptions to this rule, including Catholic AMBASD nurse Ave Bruzzichesi.

6. Rey García, *Stars for Spain*, 89.

7. Ibid., 104.

8. Barsky Tribute Dinner pamphlet, 1967, Box 5, Folder 15, Fredericka Martin Papers, Tamiment Library, New York University, New York. [Hereafter: Martin Papers.] See also: Guerra, *La Medicina en el Exilio Republicano*, 512.

9. Fredericka Martin, "Proud within Themselves," Box 5, Folder 14, Frances Patai Papers, Tamiment Library, New York University, New York. [Hereafter: Martin, "Proud within Themselves."]

10. Martin, "Proud within Themselves," Patai Papers.

11. Ibid.; Barsky, "The Surgeon," Barsky Papers, 12.

12. Smith, *American Relief Aid and the Spanish Civil War.*

13. Barsky, "The Surgeon," Barsky Papers, 12.

14. Martin, "Proud within Themselves," Patai Papers, 7–8.

15. Smith, *American Relief Aid and the Spanish Civil War*; "Medical Expedition Will Sail For Spain," *New York Times*, 11 January 1937.

16. According to Barsky, the AMBASD's first objective was to send enough equipment and personnel to furnish and staff a seventy-five–bed hospital. Fredericka Martin remembered it as a fifty–bed hospital. Martin suggested that it was only after the group began receiving unsolicited offers from interested volunteers that it considered sending personnel.

17. Smith, *American Relief Aid and the Spanish Civil War.*

18. Martin, "Proud within Themselves," Patai Papers.

19. Smith, *American Relief Aid and the Spanish Civil War.*

20. Rey García, *Stars for Spain*, 90.

21. Martin Papers, Box 14, Folder 17: "Two Years of American Aid to Spain."

22. Other names include: C.E.A. Winslow, Yale University; Howard Naffsiger, University of California, president of the American College of Surgeons; Anton J. Carlson, Chicago University; Haven Emerson, Columbia; David J. Davis, University of Illinois; E. C. Rosenow, Mayo Clinic; Bela Schic, Mt. Sinai Hospital; and Florence Sabin, Rockefeller Institute.

23. Eugene Perry Link, *The Social Ideas of American Physicians (1776–1976): Studies in the Humanitarian Tradition of Medicine* (London: Associated University Presses, 1992), 225–237.

24. Quoted in ibid., 144.

25. Guerra's *La Medicina en el Exilio Republicano* offers a rare and valuable biographical profile of American medical personnel, 511–535.

26. Helen Freeman, Questionnaire, Box 8, Folder 7, Martin Papers.

27. Ave Bruzzichesi, "I Was a Catholic Nurse in Loyalist Spain," Box 5, Folder 24, Martin Papers.

28. Zachary Stadt, Questionnaire, Box 12, Folder 2, Martin Papers.

29. Sana Goldblatt, Questionnaire, Box 8, Folder 17, Martin Papers.

30. Nurses Hilda Bell Roberts, May Levine, and Hermine Hartmann trace their knowledge of the AMBASD and decision to apply to having read about the AMBASD's work.

31. Seventeen of thirty-two respondents cited friends or professional colleagues as their source for learning of the AMBASD and influences on their decision to apply.

32. Eric R. Smith, "New York's Aid to the Spanish Republic," in *Facing Fascism: New York and the Spanish Civil War,* ed. Peter N. Carroll and James D. Fernández (New York: New York University Press, 2007).

33. Quoted in Carroll, *Odyssey of the Abraham Lincoln Brigade*, 69.

34. Ray Harris Marantz, Questionnaire, Box 8, Folder 38, Martin Papers.

35. Patai, "Heroines of the Good Fight," 83–85. Patai's demographic summaries should be considered in light of the limited number of primary accounts she cites. Drawing her research from the Martin Papers, her assertions appear based on three unpublished memoirs and eight personal interviews with surviving nurses.

36. Interview Transcript, Celia Greenspan, Julia Newman Papers, Tamiment Library, New York University, New York.

37. Ibid., 1–52.

38. I.J. Rosenbaum to Martin, 18 April 1975, Box 11, Folder 19, Martin Papers.

39. John L. Simon, Questionnaire, Box 11, Folder 38, Martin Papers.

40. Hank Rubin, *Spain's Cause Was Mine: A Memoir of an American Medic in the Spanish Civil War* (Carbondale, IL: Southern Illinois University Press, 1997).

41. The editors of Neugass's account identify "Marty" and "Berny" as Martin Grumet and Bernard Gerber. James Neugass, *War Is Beautiful: An American Ambulance Driver in the Spanish Civil War,* ed. Peter N. Carroll and Peter Glazer (New York: New Press, 2008), 7.

42. Barsky, "The Surgeon," Barsky Papers, 14.

43. Ibid., 14.

44. Ibid., 15–16.

45. Ibid., 15–16.

46. Quoted in Neugass, *War Is Beautiful.*

47. The manuscript itself developed a story of its own. Lost for over fifty years, a copy that Neugass had sent to a friend for editorial comments was found in 2000, and published as the memoir *War Is Beautiful* in 2008.

48. Neugass, *War Is Beautiful*, 9.

49. Ibid., 23.

50. Albert Byrne to Martin, undated, Box 5, Folder 30, Martin Papers.

51. Jack Klein, Questionnaire, Box 9, Folder 38, Martin Papers.

52. Eugenia Grunsky, Questionnaire, Box 8, Folder 33, Martin Papers.

53. Of thirty-two respondents, twelve checked both "political" and "humanitarian" as motivations. Eleven checked neither, but almost all of these cited a mix of both reasons in the explanation that followed. Two checked only "political" and three checked only "humanitarian."

54. Fontaine Mardfin, Questionnaire, Box 7, Folder 30, Martin Papers.

55. Irene Goldin Spiegel, Questionnaire, Box 8, Folder 18, Martin Papers.

56. Morris Kornblum, Questionnaire, Box 9, Folder 39, Martin Papers.

57. Josep L. Barona Vilar, "The Rockefeller Foundation, Social Policies and Public Health in Spain, 1920–1939," in *American Foundations and the European Welfare States* (Odense: University Press of Southern Denmark, 2013), 33–57; María Isabel Del Cura and Rafael Huertas, *Alimentación y Enfermedad En Tiempos De Hambre, España, 1937–1947* (Madrid: Consejo Superior de Investigaciones Científicas, 2007).

58. Barona Vilar, "The Rockefeller Foundation, Social Policies and Public Health in Spain."

59. The relationship between the Rockefeller Foundation and Spain was interrupted by the Spanish Civil War, but was renewed in 1940, with requests by the new Spanish government for help assessing Spain's nutritional and public health need.

60. Watt, *Health Care and National Development in Taiwan, 1950–2000*, 5.

61. Betty L. King, "Memories of Dr. Frank Co Tui: Physician, Scientist (1897–1984)," in *Health Care and National Development in Taiwan* 1950–2000, ed. Watt., 11.

62. Sweet to Edwards, 6 March 1943, Box 53, Folder 7, UCR Records, Mudd Manuscript Library, Princeton University, Princeton.

63. Watt, *Health Care and National Development in Taiwan, 1950–2000*, 6.

64. "Dr. Farn B. Chu, 35, Physician, Is Dead," *New York Times*, 20 April 1941, 43.

65. Watt, *Health Care and National Development in Taiwan, 1950–2000*, 6.

66. Ibid., 7.

67. Watt, *Health Care and National Development in Taiwan, 1950–2000*, 7.

68. "Medicine on a Mission, A History of the American Bureau for Medical Aid to China, Inc., 1937–1954," Box 11, ABMAC Records, Rare Book and Manuscript Library, Columbia University, New York. [Hereafter: "Medicine on a Mission."]

69. "Bureau to Aid Chinese", *New York Times*, 29 November 1937; "Medics to Offer Services to Aid China's Injured," *Chicago Defender*, 11 December 1937.

70. Frank Co Tui, "Plan," 11 April 1939, ABMAC Records.

71. "Medicine on a Mission," ABMAC Records, 4.

72. Ibid., 4.

73. The United Council for Civilian Relief in China shared Dr. Frank Meleney among its leadership, along with Col. Theodore Roosevelt Jr., who presided over the organization.

74. Watt, *A Friend in Deed: ABMAC and the Republic of China, 1937–1987*, 4.

75. Ibid.

76. "Medicine on a Mission," ABMAC Records. This saying was based on a legend of the Han dynasty. "One day, the story goes, a hungry, weary traveler stopped by a stream where a poor woman was washing clothes. "Will you give me something to eat?" he asked. She went into her lowly hut and returned with a steaming bowl of rice. Silently she handed it to him. The traveler devoured the food, and promised he would repay her a thousandfold. "Nonsense!" she said. "I do not expect any recompense for a simple act of charity." But a short while later the woman received a

package of one thousand pieces of gold. They were from the hungry traveler, who had now become head of the state.

77. "Medicine on a Mission," ABMAC Records, 5.

78. Co Tui, "Plan," 11 April 1939, Box 22, ABMAC Records.

79. With the influx of Chinese immigrants to the gold fields and railroads of the mid-nineteenth century U.S., racial and cultural stereotypes kept Chinese Americans marginalized, even relative to other immigrant groups. The Chinese Exclusion Act of 1882 became the first and only law to explicitly exclude a group of a people based on ethnic origin in preventing any Chinese (irrespective of technical skill) from entering the country. The act was not repealed until 1943. Dusanka Miscevic and Peter Kwong, *Chinese Americans: The Immigrant Experience* (Southport, CT: Hugh Lauter Levin Associates, Inc., 2000); Jean Pfaelzer, *Driven Out: The Forgotten War against Chinese Americans* (Berkeley: University of California Press, 2008).

80. Miscevic and Kwong, *Chinese Americans*, 124.

81. Ibid., 126.

82. Ibid.

83. Co Tui, "An Analysis," Box 22, ABMAC Records.

84. Sweet to Edwards, 21 August 1942, Box 53, Folder 10, UCR Records.

85. "Medicine on a Mission," AMBAC Redords, 4.

86. "Alumnus Presides over Medical Advancement Program in China," *P&S Journal* 18 (1998).

87. Madeline Y. Hsu, "Befriending the Yellow Peril: Student Migration and the Warming of American Attitudes Toward Chinese, 1905–1950," in *Trans-Pacific Interactions: The United States and China, 1880–1950*, Vanessa Künnemann and Ruth Mayer (New York: Palgrave Macmillan, 2009), 113.

88. For instance, the Yale-China Association was first established in 1901 as the Yale Foreign Missionary Society. The Yale-China Association would establish the Yali Middle School (a preparatory school), the College of Yale-in-China, and Hsiang-Ya Medical College (under Hume's leadership). Similarly, Princeton-in-Asia formed initially as a group to send Princeton students to China to help staff YMCA activities in Peking. Cheng also provides a valuable overview of U.S.-China educational exchanges in: Cheng Li, "Coming Home to Teach: Status and Mobility of Returnees in China's Higher Education," in *Bridging Minds across the Pacific: U.S.-China Educational Exchanges, 1978–2003*, ed. Cheng Li (Lanham: Lexington Books, 2005).

89. Jespersen, *American Images of China*, 9.

90. Alan Hunter and Chan Kim-Kwong, *Protestantism in Contemporary China* (Cambridge: Cambridge University Press, 1993), 123.

91. Neils, *China Images in the Life and Times of Henry Luce*, 60.

92. Quoted in: Jespersen, *American Images of China*, 8.

93. Itinerary of R.K.S.L., Box 2, ABMAC Records.

94. Lee Edwards, *Missionary for Freedom: The Life and Times of Walter Judd* (New York: Paragon House, 1990).

95. "Judd, Walter Henry—Biographical Information," published online at http://bioguide.congress.gov/scripts/biodisplay.pl?index=J000278 accessed 13 December 2011.

96. See Chapter 6.

97. "Medicine on a Mission," ABMAC Records, 3.

98. Watt, *A Friend in Deed: ABMAC and the Republic of China, 1937–1987*, 2.

99. International Institute, University of California Los Angeles (UCLA), "The Dentist Who Changed World History," published online at http://www.international.ucla.edu/article.asp?parentid=2813 accessed 26 Aprril 2011.

100. Quoted in: International Institute, UCLA, "The Dentist Who Changed World History."

101. Haskell to Lim, 10 August 1938, Box 1, Folder 6, New York Public Library (NYPL) Archives, New York. A later interview with Haskell dates his involvement with the CAC from 1937 or 1938. Oliver H. Haskell, "Oriental Study Expedition Oral History Project," 1989, Claremont Graduate University.

102. Haskell, "Oriental Study Expedition Oral History Project."

103. Eleanor Thompson offers an excellent introduction to educational exchanges between China and the U.S. in the 1920s in her doctoral dissertation. Eleanor Thompson, "Social Reconstructionism: An Intellectual History of Radicalism in American Education from the Progressive Era to the New Deal" (unpublished DPhil diss., Oxford: University of Oxford, 2011).

104. Haskell, "Oriental Study Expedition Oral History Project."

105. Jerry Israel, "Carl Crow, Edgar Snow, and Shifting American Journalistic Perceptions of China," in *America Views China: American Images of China Then and Now* (Bethlehem, PA: Lehigh University Press, 1991), 149.

106. Box 2, ABMAC Records.

107. Shewmaker, *Americans and Chinese Communists*, 4.

108. Bullock, *An American Transplant*, 195.

109. Board of Directors Meeting, 26 January 1942, Box 1, Opie Papers, American Philosophical Society, Philadelphia.

Two Institutional Failure: Replacing the Red Cross?

1. "The American Red Cross and National Defense," undated, Box 91, Folder 102.02, Record Group (RG) 200, Records of the American National Red Cross, National Archives and Records Administration (NARA), College Park, MD.

2. Ibid.

3. For an introduction to the ICRC and origins of the Red Cross movement; see: David P. Forsythe, *The Humanitarians: The International Committee of the Red Cross* (Cambridge: Cambridge University Press, 2005); John F. Hutchinson, *Champions of Charity: War and the Rise of the Red Cross* (Boulder: Westview Press, 1996). For its development following World War I; see: John F. Hutchinson, "'Custodians of the

Sacred Fire': The International Committee of the Red Cross and the Postwar Reorganisation of the International Red Cross," in *International Health Organisations and Movements, 1918–1939*, ed. Weindling; Bridget Towers, "Red Cross Organisational Politics, 1918–1922: Relations of Dominance and the Influence of the United States," in *International Health Organisations and Movements, 1918–1939*, ed. Weindling.

4. Forsythe, *The Humanitarians*, 26.

5. Ibid., 20.

6. Hutchinson develops this argument further in Hutchinson, *Champions of Charity*. In the case of Great Britain; see Mark Harrison, *The Medical War: British Military Medicine in the First World War* (Oxford: Oxford University Press, 2010). For the U.S.; see Irwin, *Making the World Safe*. For China; see Caroline Reeves, "From Red Crosses to Golden Arches": China, the Red Cross, and the Hague Peace Conference, 1899 -1900," in Interactions: Transregional Perspectives on World History, ed. Jerry H. Bentley, Renate Bridenthal, and Anand A. Yang. Honolulu: University of Hawaii Press, 2005; and "The Power of Mercy: The Chinese Red Cross Society, 1900–1937" (unpublished Ph.D. diss., Cambridge, MA: Harvard University, 1998).

7. Irwin, *Making the World Safe*.

8. "Congressional Charter of the American National Red Cross," May 2007, 36 U.S.C. §§300101–300111 recodified 2007, published online at www.redcross.org/images/pdfs/charter/pdf, accessed 22 February 2011.

9. The American Red Cross, "100 Significant Dates in Red Cross History," published online at www.redcross.org/images/pdfs/charter/pdf, accessed 22 February 2011. http://www.redcross.org/museum/history/100dates.asp accessed 22 February 2011.

10. This distinction may also be found in other American wartime medical activities, such as efforts to prevent venereal disease in World War I, as discussed in Allan M. Brandt, *No Magic Bullet: A Social History of Venereal Disease in the United States Since 1880* (New York: Oxford University Press, 1985); Irwin, *Making the World Safe*.

11. For more on Wilson; see: Erez Manela, *The Wilsonian Moment: Self-Determination and the International Origins of Anticolonial Nationalism* (Oxford, 2007).

12. Max Huber, The Red Cross: Principles and Problems, 1939 -1946 (Geneva: A. Kundig, 1947).

13. Ibid., 58.

14. Hutchinson, *Champions of Charity*, 287; Hutchinson, "Custodians of the Sacred Fire; Towers, "Red Cross Organizational Politics."

15. Iriye, *China and Japan in the Global Setting* (Cambridge, MA: Harvard University Press, 1992)

16. Rosenberg, *Spreading the American Dream*, 117.

17. Curti, *American Philanthropy Abroad*.

18. Karen Lynn Brewer, "From Philanthropy to Reform: The American Red Cross in China, 1906–1930" (unpublished Ph.D. diss., Case Western Reserve University).

19. Guillaume Favre to Swift, 16 April 1937, Box 17, Folder 14, Martin Papers.

20. Favre to Swift, 16 April 1937, Box 17, Folder 14, Martin Papers.

21. "Circular 335, Red Cross Action in Spain," 31 March 1937, Box 17, Folder 16, Martin Papers.

22. Norman Davis to Arthur Hamilton, 8 December 1938, Box 17, Folder 14, Martin Papers. The American Friends Service Committee also became active in China, sending units mobile units to serve in many hard-to-reach areas of China. See Davies, *Friends Ambulance Unit.*

23. "Memorandum on ARC Activities in Spain," Box 17, Folder 14, Martin Papers.

24. Sparrow, *Warfare State*, 6–7.

25. Arthur Hamilton to Norman Davis, 4 December 1938, Box 17, Folder 14, Martin Papers.

26. "Vice President of ARC Gives His Impressions of Republican Spain," 4 December 1938, Box 17, Folder 14, Martin Papers.

27. "No Red Cross Aid to Loyalists Claim," Box 8, Folder 1, Martin Papers.

28. Stadt, "War Service in Spain, Experiences at the American Hospital," *Harvard Dental Record*, 30 October 1937, Box 12, Folder 2, Martin Papers.

29. Article, *La Vanguardia*, Box 14, Folder 3, Martin Papers.

30. Article, undated, Box 8, Folder 10, Martin Papers.

31. Rey García, *Stars for Spain*, 93.

32. "Help Us Send to the Front our Hospital Caravan to Save Lives," Box 14, Folder 17, Martin Papers.

33. Ibid.

34. Stadt, "War Service in Spain," Box 12, Folder 2, Martin Papers.

35. "Woman Physician of Houston Will Join Medical Relief Unit in Spain," *Houston Post*, Box 13, Folder 19, Martin Papers.

36. "Dr. Vanzant Returns from War-Torn Spain," *Houston Press*, 21 June 1938, Box 13, Folder 19, Martin Papers.

37. "Role and Activities of the Red Cross in Time of Civil War," Sixteenth International Red Cross Conference, London, June 1938, Box 17, Folder 16, Martin Papers. The ICRC's role in civil conflicts was revisited in 1938, without significant change.

38. Jackson, *The Spanish Republic and the Civil War*, 431.

39. "Memoranda: Cooperation of International Red Cross in Spanish Revolt," Box 17, Folder 16, Martin Papers.

40. Odier to Swift, 2 August 1937, Box 17, Folder 14, Martin Papers.

41. "Reduction of Activities in Spain," 7 February 1938, Box 17, Folder 16, Martin Papers.

42. James T. Nicholson to Davis, 14 July 1939, Box 87, Folder 41, RG 200, Records of the American National Red Cross.

43. Huber, *The Red Cross*, 94–95.

44. "Chinese Casualties Estimated at 800,000," *New York Times*, 17 November 1937, 4.

45. "Chinese Will Win, Missionaries Say," *New York Times*, 1 September 1938, 11; "1942 Directory Red Cross Operations in China," Box 1395, Folder 985.3, RG 200, Records of the American National Red Cross.

46. Evert Barger and Philip Wright, "Summary of Reports on a Survey of Red Cross Work in the Northwest," July 1941, Box 22, ABMAC Records.

47. Ibid.

48. Huber, *The Red Cross*, 94–95.

49. Reeves, "From Red Crosses to Golden Arches."

50. Ibid., 93.

51. Ibid., 95.

52. "Red Cross to Accept Relief Funds," *Christian Science Monitor*, 3 September 1937, 2.

53. "For Relief in War Zone," *The Sun*, 5 September 1937, 3; "Red Cross Here to Aid Chinese," *Atlanta Constitution*, 12 September 1937, 2A.

54. "China Sufferers to get $100,000 Red Cross Aid," *Washington Post*, 30 September 1937, 7.

55. Dulles, *The American Red Cross*, 341.

56. "Red Cross Orders Drugs to Aid China's Wounded," *Washington Post*, 2 October 1937, 4; "Red Cross Equips Chinese Hospitals," *New York Times*, 3 October 1937, 32; "Princess Aids China Relief," *Los Angeles Times*, 20 October 1937, 2A.

57. G. Canby Robinson, "Letter to the Editor," *The Sun*, 24 September 1937, 12; "Chinese Restaurants Here Give for Chinese Relief," *The Sun*, 17 October 1937, 3.

58. "Chinese Given Fund Japanese Spurned," *The Sun*, 22 January 1937, 5. Dr. Robinson had a personal interest in China after having spent time at the PUMC.

59. "Roosevelt Backs Fund to Aid China," *New York Times*, 25 January 1938, 8; "Red Cross Seeking Million for China," *Atlanta Constitution*, 25 January 1938, 19; "Roosevelt Appeals for Funds to Help Chinese Civilians," *The Sun*, 25 January 1938, 1; "$1,000,000 in Chinese Relief Asked," *Washington Post*, 25 January 1938, XI; "China Relief Fund Urged," *Los Angeles Times*, 25 January 1938, 14; "President Roosevelt Asks for $1,000,000 to Aid War Sufferers," *Chicago Daily Tribune*, 25 January 1938, 5.

60. Of this, $130,000 had come directly from the ARC national treasury, while $51,000 had come from public donations.

61. "Roosevelt Backs Fund to Aid China," The American Advisory Committee was a group of American residents in China appointed by U.S. Ambassador Nelson T. Johnson, drawing largely from American business and missionary communities.

62. "$1,000,000 for Chinese Relief Asked"; "The Red Cross Appeal," *New York Times*, 26 January 1938, 22; "Red Cross Aid for China," *Washington Post*, 26 January 1938, 8.

63. "Clergy Asked to Aid China Relief Fund," *Hartford Courant*, 30 January 1938, 3; "Mrs. Roosevelt to Aid China Fund," *New York Times*, 1 February 1938; "Mrs. Roosevelt to Make Radio Plea for China," *Washington Post*, 1 February 1938, X24; "Fund Drive Postponed," *New York Times*, 30 January 1938, 33.

64. Cannon Papers, Box 40, Folder 521: Letter to Franklin D. Roosevelt, 16 March 1938.

65. "$5,000,000 for China Sought in Congress," *New York Times*, 26 January 1938, 11.

66. "Red Cross to Meet in D.C. Next Year; Urges China Help," *Washington Post*, 6 May 1938, X3.

67. "Davis Pleads Here for Chinese Fund," *New York Times*, 17 May 1938, 14.

68. "China Relief Drive Sped," *Los Angeles Times*, 6 May 1938, 3.

69. "China Relief Drive Ended," *New York Times*, 16 June 1938, 9.

70. Dulles, *The American Red Cross*, 342.

71. Letter to Franklin D. Roosevelt, 16 March 1938, Box 40, Folder 521, Cannon Papers.

72. I. M. K. Colchester, "Red Cross," *Hartford Courant*, 26 April 1938, 8.

73. "ARC Activities in China," Box 1394, Folder 985.08, RG 200, Records of the American National Red Cross.

74. "China Relief Drive Ended," *New York Times*, 16 June 1938, 9.

75. "Memo on Need for Personnel and Training," 31 October 1941, Box 22, ABMAC Records.

76. Caroline Reeves, "History of the Chinese Red Cross: Part II," China Beat, http://www.thechinabeat.org/?p=119, last updated 20 May 2008, accessed 22 February 2011. For a more complete history of the Chinese Red Cross, see: Reeves, "Power of Mercy.

77. "Memorandum on the Chinese Red Cross Medical Relief Corps," 5 March 1941, Box 42, Folder 545, Cannon Papers.

78. Ibid.

79. "Memo on Need for Personnel and Training," undated, Box 22, ABMAC Records.

80. Horace W. Davenport, *Robert Kho-Seng Lim, 1897–1969* (Washington D.C.: The National Academies Press, 1980), 283.

81. Lim's mother was reportedly one of the first Chinese women to be educated in the United States. Davenport, *Robert Kho-Seng Lim*, 286.

82. Ibid., 291.

83. Ibid., 291.

84. Cannon Papers, Box 41, Folder 533: Letter to Robert Littell, 28 April 1939.

85. Benison, Barger, and Wolfe, "Walter B. Cannon and the Mystery of Shock."

86. Josep Barona Vilar, "Negrín medico fisiólogo," in *Juan Negrín Médico y Jefe de Gobierno, 1892–1956* (Madrid: Minesterio de Cultura, SECC, 2006). For more on Negrín; see: Gabriel Jackson, *Juan Negrín: Spanish Republican War Leader* (Sussex: Sussex Academic Press, 2010).

87. The *Laboratorio de Fisiología General* was founded in 1916 by the *Junta para Ampliación de Estudios e Investigaciones Cientificas*, or JAE.

88. Elin L. Wolfe, Clifford A. Barger, and Saul Benison, *Walter B. Cannon: Science and Society* (Cambridge, MA: Harvard University Press, 2000), 338.

89. Fairbank, a specialist in Chinese history, later joined the OSS (U.S. precursor of the Central Intelligence Agency) to work in China. Maochun Yu, *OSS in China: Prelude to Cold War* (Annapolis: Naval Institute Press, 2011).

90. Wolfe, Barger, and Benison, *Walter B. Cannon: Science and Society*, 333.

91. Lim to Cannon, 13 April 1938, Box 40, Folder 517, Cannon Papers.

92. Ibid.

93. Cannon to Franklin D. Roosevelt, 24 March 1938, Box 40, Folder 521, Cannon Papers. Cannon reported that the Chinese Red Cross had donated more than $1,500,000 "for the welfare of our people."

94. Karl T. Compton to Franklin D. Roosevelt, 16 March 1938, Box 40, Folder 521, Cannon Papers.

95. Franklin D. Roosevelt to Cannon, 26 March 1938, Box 40, Folder 521, Cannon Papers.

96. Wolfe, Barger, and Benison, *Walter B. Cannon: Science and Society*, 487.

97. Co Tui, "Plan," 11 April 1939, Box 22, ABMAC Records.

98. Certificate, 1 July 1940, Box 22, ABMAC Records.

99. L. S. Woo to Co Tui, 3 August 1944, Box 22, ABMAC Records.

100. Edwards to Sweet, 13 February 1943, Box 53, Folder 7, USC Records.

101. "Excerpt from National Herald," 5 February 1943, Box 53, Folder 7, USC Records.

102. Phillips F. Greene to Allen, 26 May 1942, Box 1, ABMAC Records.

103. "Confidential Report on EMSTS," 1943, Box 53, Folder 7, USC Records; Edwards to Sweet, 14 January 1943, Box 53, Folder 7, USC Records.

104. Haskell to Lim, 10 August 1938, Box 1, Folder 6, UCR Records.

105. Ibid.

106. Lim to Haskell, 26 September 1938, Box 1, Folder 6, UCR Records.

107. Ibid.

108. Lim to Haskell, 5 September 1938, Box 1, Folder 6, UCR Records.

109. "Report of the 29th Unit at Yenan," February to September 1938, Box 1, Folder 6, UCR Records.

110. Lim to Haskell, 2 October 1938, Box 1, Folder 6, UCR Records.

111. See Chapter 2.

112. Ernest J. Swift to Cannon, 10 April 1940, Box 41, Folder 538, Cannon Papers; Box 1395, Folder 985.6, RG 200, Records of the American National Red Cross.

113. Box 1395, Folder 985.6, RG 200, Records of the American National Red Cross.

114. Swift to Cannon, 10 April 1940, Box 41, Folder 538, Cannon Papers; Swift to Co Tui, 12 October 1940, Box 41, Folder 538, Cannon Papers.

115. Box 1395, Folder 985.408, RG 200, Records of the American National Red Cross. Baker had a long history of service in China (including work with the ARC), and Wesselius had worked with the ARC in WWI before assisting domestic operations over the course of the 1920s. "Wisconsin Man Builds Good Roads to End China's Famines," *Milwaukee Journal*, 17 July 1921, 7; "Hialeah Relief Chief Arrives," *Miami Daily News*, 3 October 1926, 9.

116. "Memorandum on the Chinese Red Cross Medical Relief Corps," 5 March 1941, Box 42, Folder 545, Cannon Papers.

117. "Shipments," 30 November 1941, Box 1395, Folder 985.3, RG 200, Records of the National American Red Cross.

118. "1942 Directory," Box 1395, Folder 985.3, RG 200, Records of the National American Red Cross.

119. Part of the ABMAC's increasing distance from the Medical Relief Corps may have also been a result of the funding difficulties facing the UCR after the controversy surrounding Lim's leadership and the reorganization of the CRC.

120. Letter to Co Tui, 8 August 1941, Box 22, ABMAC Records; Lim to Greene, 11 November 1941, Box 22, ABMAC Records.

121. "Minutes of Meeting of Committee on Army Medical Administration and Chinese Red Cross in China," 26 November 1945, Box 6, ABMAC Records.

122. Gordon Stiffler Seagrave, *Burma Surgeon* (London: V. Gollancz Ltd., 1944); Donovan Webster, *The Burma Road: The Epic Story of One of World War II's Most Remarkable Endeavours* (London: Macmillan, 2003).

123. Report, 9 January 1945, Box 1395, Folder 985.408, RG 200, Records of the American National Red Cross.

124. Ibid.

125. Lim to Roger S. Greene, 11 November 1941, Box 22, ABMAC Records.

126. Box 1395, Folder 985.408, RG 200, Records of the American National Red Cross.

127. Ibid.

128. Weindling, *International Health Organisations and Movements, 1918–1939.*

129. Brewer, "From Philanthropy to Reform: The American Red Cross in China, 1906–1930." Jones, "Confronting Calamity."

Three Defining Aid: Private Interests Meet the State

1. R.S., "Memorandum," 10 December 1936, Box 627, RG 59, General Records of the Department of State.

2. Cannon to Hull, 31 December 1936, Box 14, Folder 19, Martin Papers.

3. Ibid.

4. John Hickerson to Cannon, 9 January 1937, Box 14, Folder 19, Martin Papers.

5. Licenses for personal armored cars were refused, while ambulances were allowed as non-military equipment. Folder 3, Box 14, Martin Papers.

6. J.J.S. to Mrs. Shipley, 22 January 1937, Box 627, RG 59, General Records of the Department of State.

7. Ibid.

8. Perkins to Secretary of State, 22 January 1937, Box 14, Folder 3, Martin Papers.

9. Ibid.

10. Perkins to State Department, Box 14, Folder 3, Martin Papers.

11. Telegram, State Department to American Consul, 26 February 1937, Box 14, Folder 3, Martin Papers.

12. Telegram, Roger Chase to Cordell Hull, 13 February 1937, Box 14, Folder 19, Martin Papers.

13. Passport Division to James Clement Dunn, 16 February 1937, Box 14, Folder 19, Martin Papers.

14. "U.S. Bars Americans From Going to Spain; Members of Ambulance Units Are Included," *New York Times*, Box 14, Folder 19, Martin Papers.

15. Roger Baldwin to AMBASD, 15 March 1937, Box 7, Folder 29, Martin Papers.

16. State Department to Joint Committee of Physicians, 22 Mar 1937, Box 7, Folder 29, Martin Papers.

17. Telegram, Hull to American Consul, 19 March 1937, Box 627, RG 59, General Records of the Department of State.

18. Wilbur J. Carr to Maxwell Blake, 1 March 1937, Box 627, RG 59, General Records of the Department of State.

19. Perkins to State Department, 20 April 1937, Box 14, Folder 3, Martin Papers.

20. Ibid.

21. Douglas Flood, "Passports of American Citizens Serving as Volunteers in the Spanish Government Forces," 20 July 1937; A.J.N., "Memorandum for the file," Box 627, RG 59, General Records of the Department of State.

22. Rey García, *Stars for Spain*, 92.

23. Ibid., 93.

24. Doctor Serving at Spanish Frontier Tells of War Horror, Human Suffering," *Bergen Evening Record*, 12 August 1937, Box 8, Folder 10, Martin Papers; "Red Cross Vanishing," *New York Sun*, 19 July 1937, Box 2, Folder 13, Barsky Papers.

25. Taithe, "Red Cross Flag," 26–27.

26. Mark Harrison, "Medicine and the Management of Modern Warfare," *History of Science* 34 (1996): 379–410.

27. "Tells of Raids on Red Cross, Dr. Barsky, Home From Spain Says the Symbol No Longer Gives Immunity in War," *New York World Telegram*, 19 July 1937, Box 2, Folder 13, Barsky Papers.

28. "Fascist Airman Bomb Hospitals, Says U.S. Doctor," *New York Post*, 19 July 1937, Box 2, Folder 13, Barsky Papers.

29. Neugass, *War Is Beautiful*, 167.

30. Ibid., 210.

31. Smith, *American Relief Aid and the Spanish Civil War.*

32. Smith's research confirms the latter, as reported in January 1937. Smith suggests that such political infighting worked against relief efforts by raising doubts both among Spanish Republican officials and the U.S. public. Ibid.

33. Smith, *American Relief Aid and the Spanish Civil War.*

34. Jespersen, *American Images of China*, 49.

35. Hugh Thomas, *The Spanish Civil War,* 4th ed. (London: Penguin, 2003), 854.

36. Neils, *China Images in the Life and Times of Henry Luce*, 61.

37. These included Pearl S. Buck (novelist), William C. Bullitt (former U.S. ambassador to the U.S.S.R.), Paul G. Hoffman (chairman of the Studebaker corporation

and future Marshall Plan administrator), Thomas W. Lamont (Morgan House banker), John D. Rockefeller, III (of the Rockefeller Foundation), Col. Theodore Roosevelt, Jr., David O. Selznick (producer of *Gone with the Wind*), and Wendell L. Willkie (1940 Republican presidential candidate). James G. Blaine (president of the Marine Midland Trust Company) served as UCR's first chairman.

38. Jespersen, *American Images of China*, 48.

39. Ibid., 47.

40. Quoted in Neils, *China Images in the Life and Times of Henry Luce*, 72.

41. Jespersen, *American Images of China*, 50.

42. Quoted in ibid., 56.

43. Ibid., 57.

44. Jespersen, *American Images of China*, 55.

45. Ibid., 48.

46. Sweet to Edwards, 6 July 1942, Box 53, Folder 10, USC Records.

47. Sweet to Edwards, 6 July 1942, Box 53, Folder 10, USC Records.

48. Helen Kennedy Stevens was the ABMAC's executive director at the time.

49. ABMAC Bulletin, Vol. III, No. II, December 1941–January 1942, Box 1, Opie Papers.

50. Claude Forkner's involvement in the China Aid Council seems to have arisen through the affiliated American Committee for Chinese War Orphans. His involvement is somewhat surprising, as Forkner was much more a part of the Rockefeller contingent that joined forces with ABMAC. However, less than a year after the China Aid Council joined UCR, Forkner resigned, citing his rising awareness "during the past six or eight months . . . of the fact that my ideas and ideals as they relate to the work of our organization are not in accord with those of the majority of the active members of the executive committee." Forkner remained active in aid to China through other avenues, directing the China Medical Board during the war, serving as a consultant to the surgeon general of the U.S. Army in the China-Burma-India theater under Generals Stilwell and Wedemeyer, and acting as advisor to a commission on medical education in China sponsored by the Chinese Ministry of Education. "Information Requested from China Agencies," undated, Box 32, Folder 9, USC Records; Forkner to CAC, 13 November 1941, Box 32, Folder 5, USC Records.

51. As UCR evolved, however, and the ABMAC increasingly became the dominant "medical" agency under UCR, the CAC increasingly played up its activities in supporting child welfare through Soong Ching Ling's "warphanages" for Chinese war orphans. "Report on Requests for Second Stage Allotments Under UCR," September 1941, Box 32, Folder 5, USC Records.

52. R.B. Shipley to Somerset A. Owen, 18 August 1937, Box 606, RG 59, General Records of the Department of State.

53. Hull to Embassy (Nanking), 27 September 1937, Box 606, RG 59, General Records of the Department of State.

54. Harold J. Seymour, *Design for Giving: The Story of the National War Fund, Inc., 1943–1947* (New York: Harper & Brothers, 1947), 3.

55. Ibid., 3.

56. Franklin D. Roosevelt, "Executive Order 9205 Establishing the President's War Relief Control Board," July 25, 1942, published online by *The American Presidency Project*, ed. Gerhard Peters and John T. Woolley, http://www.presidency.ucsb.edu/ws/?pid=16287 accessed 20 June 2013.

57. David McKean, Peddling Influence: Thomas "Tommy the Cork" Corcoran and the Birth of Modern Lobbying (Hanover, NH: Steerforth, 2005).

58. D.M. Corcoran to Bank of China, 30 April 1941, Box 2, Frederic A. Delano Papers, Franklin Delano Roosevelt Presidential Library, Hyde Park.

59. CDS to Secretary of State, 27 May 1941, Box 2, Delano Papers.

60. Soong, educated at Harvard, was also Chiang's minister of finance, personal banker, and brother-in-law.

61. "Conference on the Present Medical Situation in China," 15 June 1946, Box 1, ABMAC Records.

62. Chinese Supply Commission to Harry L. Hopkins, 5 July 1944, Box 173, Harry L. Hopkins Papers, Franklin Delano Roosevelt Presidential Library, Hyde Park.

63. Those in attendance included: Edward C. Carter (Institute of Pacific Relations); Marshall Balfour (Rockefeller Foundation); David Bruce (ARC); Walter B. Cannon (Harvard); Charles Corbett (Church Committee for China Relief); Frank Co Tui (China Defense Supplies, Inc.); Claude Forkner (Cornell); B.A. Garside (UCR Executive Director); Ralph G. Hubbell (ARC); Edwin C. Lobenstine (CMB); W.W. Lockwood (American Committee for International Studies); L.M. Mitchell (ARC); Eugene L. Opie (Cornell); Harry Price (China Defense Supplies, Inc.); Philip E. Ryan (ARC); Christopher Sharman (AFSC); Donald D. Van Slyke (Rockefeller Institute); Admiral Harry E. Yarnell (U.S. Navy); Mr. Robert W. Barnett (UCR).

64. "Confidential Report," 31 July 1941, Box 1, Folder 1, ABMAC Records.

65. Sweet to Edwards, 5 February 1943, Box 53, Folder 7, USC Records.

66. Seymour, *Design for Giving*, 38.

67. Already in 1942 this pattern had been expanded to a state level in Alabama and Rhode Island.

68. Seymour, *Design for Giving*, 4.

69. Ibid., 9.

70. "Your Gift Circles the Globe," Box 38, Folder 3, USC Records; "These Next Six Months Will Tell," 1 August 1945, Box 38, Folder 3, USC Records.

71. Seymour, *Design for Giving*, 14.

72. Ibid., 20.

73. Sparrow, *Warfare State*, 6–7.

74. Edwards to Sweet, 8 May 1943, Box 53, Folder 6, USC Records.

75. See Chapter 2.

76. Edwards to Sweet, 14 April 1943, Box 53, Folder 6, USC Records.

77. 18 May 1944, Box 1, Folder 1, ABMAC Records.

78. Binder, Box 1, Folder 1, ABMAC Records.

79. Edwards to Sweet, 14 April 1943, Box 53, Folder 6, USC Records.

80. Sweet to Edwards, 6 January 1943, Box 53, Folder 7, USC Records.

81. Binder, Box 1, Folder 1, ABMAC Records.

82. Ibid.

83. Mr. Lauchlin Currie to President Roosevelt, 15 March 1941, *Foreign Relations of the United States, 1944, Vol. VI, China* (Washington: GPO, 1947), 94.

84. General Ho to Sweet, 22 July 1945, Box 51, Folder 9, USC Records.

85. Neugass, *War Is Beautiful*, 235.

86. Ibid., 244.

87. Ibid., 63.

Four American Medical Volunteers in Spain

1. Martin, "Proud within Themselves," Patai Papers, 3.

2. Barsky and Rackley to AMBASD, 20 April 1937, Box 5, Folder 17, Martin Papers.

3. "Report on the Health Mission in Spain," Box 14, Folder 13, Martin Papers.

4. Quoted in Coni, *Medicine and Warfare*, 153.

5. Josep Lluís Barona Vilar, *Salud, Enfermedad y Muerte: La Sociedad Valenciana Entre 1833 y 1939* (Valencia: Institucio Alfons El Magnanim. 2002), 348.

6. Barsky, "The Surgeon," Barsky Papers, 22.

7. Ibid.

8. Navarro Carballo, *La Sanidad En Las Brigadas Internacionales*, 79–80; Massons, *Historia De La Sanidad Militar Española*, 338. Navarro Carballo cites thirty-two different hospitals in Madrid itself; Massons claims there were thirty-seven. Among these, Navarro Carballo lists two "Hospital Auxiliar de la Cruz Roja."

9. Navarro Carballo, *La Sanidad En Las Brigadas Internacionales*, 80.

10. Barsky, "The Surgeon," Barsky Papers, 22.

11. Lini (Fuhr) De Vries, "Up from the Cellar," Box 7, Folders 26–28, Martin Papers.

12. Barsky, "The Surgeon," Barsky Papers, 18.

13. Martin, "Proud within Themselves," Patai Papers, 5–6.

14. Ibid., 5–6.

15. Coni, *Medicine and Warfare*, 133.

16. Ibid., 132.

17. Carl Geiser Papers, Tamiment Library, New York University, New York; Letter to Mug, 28 August 1937, Box 1, Folder 4, Paul Wendorf Papers, Tamiment Library, New York University, New York; to Mother and Sister, 18 September 1937, Box 1, Folder 2, Vincent Lossowski Papers; Letter to Ruth, 22 December 1937 and 26 December 1937, Box 1, Folder 6, Jacob Shafran Papers.

18. Letter to Impy, 16 October 1937, Box 1, Folder 6, Geiser Papers.

19. Letter to Impy, 29 October 1937, Box 1, Folder 6; Letter to Impy, 5 November 1937, Box 1, Folder 7; Letter to Impy, 5 December 1937, Box 1, Folder 1, Geiser Papers.

20. Letter to Impy, 8 November 1937, Box 1, Folder 6, Geiser Papers.

21. Mitch to Ruth Goldstein, 22 September 1938, Box 1, Folder 17, Shafran.

22. Navarro Carballo, *La Sanidad en Las Brigadas Internacionales*, 77.

23. Massons, *Historia de la Sanidad Militar Española*, 332.

24. Navarro Carballo, *La Sanidad en Las Brigadas Internacionales*, 82.

25. Barsky and Rackley to AMBASD, 20 April 1937, Box 5, Folder 17, Martin Papers.

26. Eloesser to Bob Miner, 30 March 1938, Box 7, Folder 11, Martin Papers.

27. Navarro Carballo, *La Sanidad en Las Brigadas Internacionales*, 141; Massons, *Historia de la Sanidad Militar Española*, 338. Almost 18 percent of doctors within the SSI were women—a much higher concentration than within the profession as a whole at the time.

28. Coni, *Medicine and Warfare*, 131.

29. Martin, "Proud within Themselves," Patai Papers, 7.

30. Navarro Carballo, *La Sanidad en Las Brigadas Internacionales*, 104.

31. Ibid., 83.

32. Coni, *Medicine and Warfare*, 133.

33. Mary Louise Platkin, Diary, 26 July 1937, Box 11, Folder 5, Martin Papers.

34. The next highest donor was Switzerland, contributing 315,000 francs, followed by France, contributing 239,500 francs. Barona Vilar, 345.

35. International Brigade volunteers donated four million pesetas to the SSI during the war. One ambulance driver reported on SRI donations from hospitals arising as a self-sentencing penalty in trials of patients for drunkenness. Navarro Carballo, *La Sanidad en Las Brigadas Internacionales*, 140; Neugass, *War Is Beautiful*, 14–15.

36. Navarro Carballo, *La Sanidad en Las Brigadas Internacionales*, 98–99; Coni, *Medicine and Warfare*, 135.

37. Coni, *Medicine and Warfare*, 135.

38. "Carnet Militar," Eugenia Grunsky, Box 8, Folder 26, Martin Papers.

39. Interview, Dr. Jose Fuche Alvarez, 21 May 1971, Box 14, Folder 9, Martin Papers.

40. Ibid.

41. Coni, *Medicine and Warfare*, 134.

42. Navarro Carballo, *La Sanidad en Las Brigadas Internacionales*, 132.

43. Coni, *Medicine and Warfare*, 135.

44. Ibid., 136.

45. Irving Busch, "With Our American Hospitals," *The Volunteer for Liberty*, Box 5, Folder 26, Martin Papers.

46. Navarro Carballo, *La Sanidad en Las Brigadas Internacionales*, 102.

47. Ibid., 103.

48. CSI to AMBASD, 26 April 1938, Box 5, Folder 17, Martin Papers.

49. Barsky, "The Surgeon," Barsky Papers, 27–28.

50. Ibid., 28.

51. The shortage of food was one of the greatest challenges to physicians in Spain, both in civil and military hospitals. "Account of Dr. Barney Malbin," Box 10, Folder 3, Martin Papers.

52. Barsky, "The Surgeon," Barsky Papers, 32.

53. A "skeleton staff" of doctors and nurses was left in Romeral to look after the handful of patients who could not yet be moved until they could be evacuated. These included Drs. Perez and Bloom, alongside nurses Lini De Vries and Ray Harris. Mildred Rackley to Martin, 5 August 1971, Box 11, Folder 11, Martin Papers.

54. Rackley to Martin, 5 August 1971, Box 11, Folder 11, Martin Papers.

55. Ibid.

56. Rackley to Martin, 5 August 1971, Box 11, Folder 11, Martin Papers.

57. Telge, "A Year of Heroic Work," *Ayuda Médica Internacional (AMI)*, Box 8, Folder 11, Martin Papers.

58. Barsky and Rackley to AMBASD, 20 April 1937, Box 5, Folder 17, Martin Papers.

59. Coni, *Medicine and Warfare*, 129.

60. Busch, "With Our American Hospitals," *The Volunteer for Liberty*, Box 5, Folder 26, Martin Papers.

61. Letter to Mom and Sis, 6 October 1937, Box 1, Folder 2, Lossowski Papers. Photos of the interior of the hospital—including canteen, library, and wards—at Benicasim can be found at the Imperial War Museum's collection of Spanish Civil War photographs.

62. Luba Brisker, "Recollections of My Almost 2 Years in Spain during the Spanish War 1936–1939," Box 5, Folder 22, Martin Papers.

63. "A Year of Heroic Work," Box 8, Folder 11, Martin Papers. An exterior photo of the hospital at Murcia can also be found in the Imperial War Museum collection.

64. Ibid.

65. Albert E. Cowdrey, *Fighting for Life: American Military Medicine in World War II* (New York: Free Press, 1994), 7; William Wiesmann, Nicole Draghic, and John A. Parrish, "Advances in Modern Combat Casualty Care with a Vision to the Future," in *War and Medicine*, ed. Wellcome Trust (London: Black Dog, 2008), 231.

66. Abraham Friedman to AMBASD, 10 September 1937, Box 8, Folder 9, Martin Papers; Ena Ferwerda to Martin, Box 7, Folder 22, Martin Papers. The AMBASD also explored instigating an anti-malarial campaign with funding from the Rockefeller Foundation, although these plans never seem to have gotten off the ground. Letter to Reissig, 18 February 1938, Box 17, Folder 22, Martin Papers.

67. Fontaine to Martin, 30 January 1969, Box 7, Folder 24; Radio Interview, Norman Rintz, February 1938, Box 16, Folder 36, Martin Papers.

68. Abraham Friedman, "The Southern Front," *AMI*, Box 5, Folder 26, Martin Papers.

69. Neugass, *War Is Beautiful*, 117–118.

70. Ibid., 116.

71. Radio Interview, Rintz, Box 16, Folder 36, Martin Papers. For a vivid account of this episode; see also Neugass, *War Is Beautiful*, 96.

72. Coni, *Medicine and Warfare*, 130.

73. Neugass, *War Is Beautiful*, 261.

74. Ibid., 220.

75. Abraham Ettelson, "The American Neurosurgical Unit in Spain," *AMI*, No. 10, 1 March 1938, Box 7, Folder 19, Martin Papers.

76. Ibid.

77. Barsky and Rackley to AMBASD, 20 April 1937, Box 5, Folder 17, Martin Papers.

78. John Posner, "Oral Surgeon in the Spanish Civil War," *Oral Hygiene*, June 1942, Box 11, Folder 7, Martin Papers.

79. Klein, Questionnaire, Box 9, Folder 37, Martin Papers.

80. Frances Vanzant to Rackley, 21 April 1938, Box 15, Folder 14, Martin Papers.

81. Ibid.

82. Bruzzichesi, "I Was a Catholic Nurse," Box 5, Folder 24, Martin Papers.

83. "Account of Dr. Barney Malbin," Box 10, Folder 3, Martin Papers.

84. Harris B. Shumaker, *Leo Eloesser, M.D.: Eulogy for a Free Spirit* (New York: Philosophical Library, 1982), 181; Klein, Questionnaire, Box 9, Folder 37, Martin Papers.

85. Barney Malbin, "Typhoid Fever Occurring in Immunized Persons," *Journal of the American Medical Association* 115 (1940): 33–36.

86. Fontaine to Martin, 19 April 1970, Box 7, Folder 24, Martin Papers.

87. De Vries, "Up from the Cellar," Box 7, Folders 26–28, Martin Papers.

88. Eloesser to AMBASD, 22 January 1938, Box 7, Folder 11, Martin Papers.

89. Leonora Temple, Questionnaire, Box 13, Folder 5, Martin Papers.

90. Dexter Waugh, "Lincoln Brigade Honors Women," *San Francisco Examiner*, 25 January 1977, Box 4, Folder 3, Patai Papers.

91. Thelma Erickson to Mother, 2 March 1938, Box 5, Folder 29, Martin Papers.

92. Neugass, *War Is Beautiful*, 167, 212.

93. Ibid., 108; Anne Taft to Martin, 2 February 1969, Box 12, Folder 11, Martin Papers.

94. Freeman, Questionnaire, Box 8, Folder 7, Martin Papers.

95. Fredericka Martin, Diary, Box 10, Folder 13, Martin Papers.

96. AMBASD, News Release, Box 6, Folder 3, Martin Papers.

97. Letter, 2–3 September, Box 1, Folder 3, Smith Papers, Tamiment Library, New York University, New York.

98. Ann Shuldiner to Martin, 12 August 1968, Box 11, Folder 34, Martin Papers.

99. Friedman, "Operating Under Flickering Flashlight to Accompaniment of Bombs," *Bergen Evening Record*, 30 March 1938, Box 8, Folder 10; Irene Goldin Spiegel to Martin, 2 February 1969, Box 8, Folder 18; Ray Harris Marantz, Radio Speech, 16 January 1938, Box 8, Folder 38, Martin Papers; "The Southern Front," *AMI*, Box 5, Folder 26, Martin Papers.

100. Letter to Ruth, 1 January 1938, Box 1, Folder 7, Shafran Papers.

101. Letter to Impy, 26 October 1937, Box 1, Folder 6, Geiser Papers.

102. Letter to Impy, 21 November 1937, Box 1, Folder 7, Geiser Papers.

103. Neugass, *War Is Beautiful*, 19.

104. S.H Abramson, "The Anglo-American Group in Benicasim," *AMI*, No. 9, 1 February 1938, Box 15, Folder 18, Martin Papers.

105. Letter to Impy, 13 December 1937, Box 1, Folder 8, Geiser Papers.

106. De Vries, "Up from the Cellar," Box 7, Folders 26–28, Martin Papers.

107. Rackley to Martin, 5 August 1971, Box 11, Folder 11, Martin Papers.

108. August Towsen to Martin, 19 August 1968, Box 13, Folder 10, Martin Papers.

109. Martin to Fontaine, 12 February 1971, Box 7, Folder 25, Martin Papers.

110. Salaria Kee O'Reilly, "While Passing Through," *Health & Medicine*4/1 (Spring 1987): 11–13.

111. Martin to Irene Goldin Spiegel, 10 September 1970, Box 8, Folder 18, Martin Papers.

112. Fontaine to Martin, 30 January 1969, Box 7, Folder 24, Martin Papers.

113. Anonymous Questionnaires, Box 11, Folder 7, Martin Papers.

114. Guerra, *La Medicina en el Exilio Republicano.*

115. "Americana Infermera," Box 11, Folder 7, Martin Papers.

116. Martin to Fontaine, 5 May 1970, Box 7, Folder 24, Martin Papers.

117. Neugass, *War Is Beautiful*, 22.

118. Toby Jensky, 17 July 1937, Box 1, Folder 1, Toby Jensky and Philip Schachter Papers.

119. Jensky, 9 May 1937 and Jensky, 17 July 1937, Box 1, Folder 1; Jensky, 11 November 1937, Box 1, Folder 1, Jensky and Schacter Papers.

120. Letter, Monica Milward, Box 8, Folder 19, Martin Papers.

121. Guerra, *La Medicina en el Exilio Republicano*, 520.

122. Thelma Erickson to Mom, 2 March 1938, Box 5, Folder 29, Martin Papers.

123. Mark Rauschwald to Martin, 11 October 1970, Box 8, Folder 11, Martin Papers.

124. Fontaine to Martin, 19 April 1970, Box 7, Folder 24; Ray Harris Marantz to Martin, Box 8, Folder 37, Martin Papers.

125. Mary Louise Platkin, Diary, 26 July 1937, Box 11, Folder 5, Martin Papers.

126. Celia Greenspan, 11 July 1937, Box 11, Folder 31, Martin Papers.

127. A.L. Cochrane to Martin, 15 July 1971, Box 14, Folder 15, Martin Papers.

128. Herbert Matthews, "Three Raids on Valencia," *New York Times*, 6 July 1938.

129. Waller, 19 August 1938, Box 13, Folder 7, Martin Papers.

130. Rebecca Schulman, Interview, Box 1, Item 66–16; Anne Taft, Interview, Box 1, Items 66-52 and 66-53, Arthur H. Landis Oral History Collection, Tamiment Library, New York University, New York.

131. Box 1, Folder 2, Wilkes Papers, Tamiment Library, New York University, New York.

132. "Guide to the Harry Wilkes Papers, 1937–1938," 2006, Tamiment Library, New York University, New York.

133. Martin added that linguistic difficulties were compounded by the "innocence and unworldliness of our most sophisticated gals which even the English with their freer sex habits shocked." Martin to Fontaine, 12 February 1971, Box 7, Folder 24, Martin Papers.

134. Martin to Spiegel, 10 September 1970, Box 8, Folder 18, Martin Papers.

135. Bruzzichesi, "I Was a Catholic Nurse," Box 5, Folder 24, Martin Papers.

136. Martin to Spiegel, 10 September 1970, Box 8, Folder 18, Martin Papers.

137. Frances Vanzant, 22 November 1937, Box 13, Folder 19, Martin Papers.

138. Ibid.

139. Julius Hene, 15 August 1937, Box 9, Folder 10, Martin Papers.

140. Josefa Andres, trans. Aelwen Wetherby, 2012; Juana Barreras Fato, trans. by Aelwen Wetherby, 2012. (Interviews conducted by Dorothy Eubanks.)

141. Barsky, "The Surgeon," Barsky Papers, 28.

142. De Vries, "Up from the Cellar," Box 6, Folders 26–28, Martin Papers.

143. Shuldiner to Martin, 12 August 1968, Box 11, Folder 34, Martin Papers.

144. Neugass, *War Is Beautiful*, 29.

145. De Vries, "Up from the Cellar," Box 6, Folders 26–28, Martin Papers; Shuldiner to Martin, 12 August 1968, Box 11, Folder 34; Ruth Davidow, Autograph Book, Box 6, Folder 10, Martin Papers.

146. Neugass, *War Is Beautiful*, 174.

147. Ibid.

148. Jose Maria Thomas, *Roosevelt and Franco During the Second World War: From the Spanish Civil War to Pearl Harbor* (New York: Palgrave Macmillan, 2008), 20.

149. Dominic Tierney, *FDR and the Spanish Civil War: Neutrality and Commitment in the Struggle That Divided America* (Durham: Duke University Press, 2007).

150. Dallek, *Franklin D. Roosevelt and American Foreign Policy*, 178–180.

151. Ibid.

152. Ibid., 122.

153. Bruzzichesi, "I Was a Catholic Nurse," Box 5, Folder 24, Martin Papers.

154. Ibid.

155. Bruzzichesi to Eloesser, 29 January 1940, Box 1, Folder 5, Patai Papers.

156. Dallek, *Franklin D. Roosevelt and American Foreign Policy*, 178–180.

Five Avenues of Aid for Americans in China

1. Letter to Co Tui, 8 August 1941, Box 22, ABMAC Records.

2. "Program of the ABMAC," 30 June 1941, Box 1, Opie Papers.

3. Minutes, Board of Directors Meeting, 26 January 1942, Box 1, Opie Papers.

4. Of four public health experts considered, negotiations were underway with Dr. Arne Barkhaus and George Bachman, while two other volunteers—Dr. Nathan Sinai and Dr. Robert Korns—were unable to accept. Surgeon Dr. Adrian Taylor had been reportedly considered, but was also unable to accept. It was unclear if Barkhaus, being born in Denmark—and married to a German-born woman—would have trouble getting a visa. Minutes, Board of Directors Meeting, 26 January 1942, Box 1, Opie Papers.

5. Agenda, Medical Committee Meeting, 24 March 1942, Box 1, Opie Papers.

6. Minutes, Medical Committee Meeting, 28 April 1942, Box 1, Opie Papers.

7. Minutes, Board of Directors Meeting, 26 January 1942, Box 1, Opie Papers.

8. Agenda, Medical Committee Meeting, 24 March 1942, Box 1, Opie Papers.

9. Wang and Cheng, "Leo Eloesser: An American Cardiothoracic Surgeon in China."

10. Report on Purchasing, Collecting, Shipping, March 1942, Box 1, Opie Papers.

11. Minutes, Board of Directors Meeting, 26 January 1942, Box 1; Agenda, Medical Committee Meeting, 24 February 1942, Box 1, Opie Papers.

12. There appears to be some disagreement over the extent to which Scudder and Drew each contributed to this project, with some arguing that Scudder had very little to do with it. Spencie Love, *One Blood: The Death and Resurrection of Charles R. Drew* (Chapel Hill: University of North Carolina Press, 1997); The Charles R. Drew Papers, Profiles in Medicine, National Library of Medicine, "Plasma for Great Britain," published online at http://profiles.nlm.nih.gov/BG/ accessed 22 May 2013.

13. The Charles R. Drew Papers, "Plasma for Great Britain."

14. Edwards to Sweet, 1 December 1943, Box 53, Folder 4, USC Records.

15. In the first group sent were Chien Lung-Yi (M.D.), C.S. Fan (M.D.), Louis de Fott, Jean Chun Liu, Luetta Chen, Ruth Derr, Adet Lin, and Betty Eng. Edwards to Sweet, 1 December 1943, Box 53, Folder 4, USC Records.

16. Edwards to Sweet, 1 December 1943, Box 53, Folder 4, USC Records.

17. Minutes, 24 October 1944, Box 1, Opie Papers.

18. Sweet to MF, 14 April 1945, Box 52, Folder 3, USC Records.

19. Scudder to Edison, 14 May 1945, Box 52, Folder 2, USC Records.

20. Sweet to Edison, 16 May 1945, Box 52, Folder 2, USC Records.

21. Ibid.

22. Agenda, Medical Committee Meeting, 24 March 1942, Box 1, Opie Papers.

23. Minutes, 27 October 1942, Box 2, Opie Papers.

24. Minutes, Medical Committee Meeting, 28 April 1942, Box 1, Opie Papers.

25. Biographical details courtesy of the research notes of Dr. Nicole Barnes, shared via e-mail 27 June 2013. Based on research conducted at Rockefeller Foundation Archives in Tarrytown, New York.

26. Agenda, Medical Committee Meeting, 24 March 1942, Box 1, Opie Papers.

27. Two other Rockefeller fellows, Dr. S.C. Chen and Mr. Jen-Chun Chang, planned to return in this group, although canceled at the last minute. Minutes, Medical Committee Meeting, 22 September 1942, Box 2, Opie Papers.

28. Agenda, Medical Committee Meeting, 24 March 1942, Box 1, Opie Papers.

29. Ibid.

30. Lin to Co Tui, 20 November 1941, Box 77, Folder 540, Rockefeller Foundation Archives, Tarrytown, New York. Courtesy of Dr. Nicole Barnes.

31. Agenda, Medical Committee Meeting, 24 March 1942, Box 1, Opie Papers.

32. Minutes, 11 January 1944, Box 2, Opie Papers.

33. This unit consisted of: J.C. Chang, Y.P. Liu (Harvard), S.C. Shen, Tsui-Mei Huang Sung, Mildred Tie, H.Y. Wang, Helena Wong, and Marion Yang. Minutes, 5 October 1943, Box 2, Opie Papers.

34. Minutes, 5 October 1943, Box 2, Opie Papers.

35. Minutes, 11 January 1944, Box 2, Opie Papers.

36. Minutes, Medical Committee Meeting, 28 April 1942, Box 1, Opie Papers.

37. Foster to parents, 27 July 1936, John B. Foster Papers, Minnesota Historical Society, Minneapolis, MN.

38. Foster to parents, 2 January 1938, Foster Papers.

39. Foster's left-wing political leanings remained unshaken and in the 1960s he became an outspoken critic of American involvement in Vietnam. He returned to China in 1974.

40. Jean Ewen, *China Nurse 1932–1939* (Toronto: McClelland and Stewart, 1981), 9.

41. Ewen, *China Nurse*, 35.

42. Ewen cites the signing as taking place in October 1936, although scholars have generally suggested that the formal agreement did not occur until later (with dates ranging from December 1936 to April 1937). Ibid., 43; Rana Mitter, *A Bitter Revolution: China's Struggle with the Modern World* (Oxford: Oxford University Press, 2004); Jonathan D. Spence, *The Search for Modern China* (New York: W.W. Norton & Company, 1990); Steve Tsang, "Chiang Kai-shek's 'Secret Deal' at Xian and the Start of the Sino-Japanese War," *Palgrave Communications* 1, published online 20 January 2015, http://www.palgrave-journals.com/articles/palcomms20143

43. Ewen, *China Nurse*, 45–46.

44. Ibid., 48.

45. It was not, however, the first. Dr. Frederic Duran I Jorda had already set up a similar service in Barcelona, although it did not cover as large an area. Stewart and Stewart, *Phoenix: The Life of Norman Bethune*.

46. Ibid., 205.

47. Allan and Gordon, *The Scalpel, the Sword*, 165.

48. Some evidence suggests that the American League for Peace and Democracy took on the bulk of these expenses. The exact relationship between this organization and the CAC is unclear, although Ewen's memoir suggests that the two were related, at least initially.

49. Shapiro, *Ma Haide.*

50. Ibid., 33.

51. Ibid., 34.

52. Ibid., 44.

53. Shapiro, *Ma Haide*, 2.

54. Sichon, "Mémoires et témoignages, Les médicins des deux guerres."

55. Ibid.

56. Dr. W. Freudmann, *Erhebet Euch! Ein Arzt Erlebt China* (Verlag, Linz-Urfahr: Neue Zeit, 1947); Fritz Jensen, *China Siegt* (Wien: Stern, 1949).

57. UCR Records, "A Guerrilla Doctor Reports from China," January 1945, Box 77, Folder 13, USC Records.

58. Mueller attributes his death to overwork and a lack of the sulfa drugs necessary to treat the disease.

59. Box 2, Folders 1–2, UCR Records.

60. Israel Epstein, *Woman in World History: Life and Times of Soong Ching Ling (Mme. Sun Yatsen)* (Beijing: Foreign Languages Press, 2004), 324.

61. Ibid., 356.

62. Ibid., 356.

63. Ibid., 357.

64. Ibid., 361.

65. Report, November 1939, Box 3, Folders 3–5, UCR Records.

66. Executive Committee Meeting, 10 March 1942, Box 1, Opie Papers.

67. Frank V. Slack to Garside, 19 March 1942, Box 53, Folder 10, USC Records.

68. Garside to Frank V. Slack, 16 March 1942, Box 53, Folder 10, USC Records.

69. Pao-Nan describes going to Calcutta for two reasons: to acquaint himself with local conditions and purchase medical supplies for the NHA, as requested by P.Z. King. He also met J.B. Grant, director of the All India Institute of Health and Public Hygiene. Pao-Nan to Frank Meleney, 26 March 1942, Box 1, Opie Papers.

70. Minutes, 5 October 1943, Box 2, Opie Papers.

71. Rockefeller funding and U.S. medical education had also contributed to King's career development in the shape of an International Health Board Fellowship to study public health at Johns Hopkins. Bullock, *An American Transplant.*

72. Sweet to Edwards, 5 February 1943, Box 53, Folder 7, USC Records.

73. Minutes, 15 September 1942, Box 2, Opie Papers.

74. Ben M. Cherrington, "The Division of Cultural Relations," *Public Opinion Quarterly* 3 (1939): 136–138.

75. "Medical Activities in China," Folder 2135, Roger S. Greene Papers, Houghton Library, Harvard University, Cambridge.

76. Greene to Grummon, 10 April 1942, Folder 778, Greene Papers.

77. Minutes, 27 October 1942, Box 2, Opie Papers.

78. Greene to Haldore Hanson, 27 November 1942, Folder 780, Greene Papers.

79. This physician was Dr. Jules Freund. Folders 788–789, Greene Papers.

80. Royal Arch Gunnison, "Construction Miracle: China's Yunnan Burma Railroad," *San Francisco Chronicle*, 27 November 1941.

81. General Ho to Sweet, 22 July 1945, Box 51, Folder 9, USC Records.

82. Forkner to Edward Carter, 20 September 1941, Box 32, Folder 5, USC Records.

83. Box 2, Folder 16, UCR Records.

84. Ibid.

85. Edwards to Sweet, 7 December 1943, Box 53, Folder 4, USC Records.

86. Sweet to Edwards, 24 April 1942, Box 53, Folder 10, USC Records.

87. Edwards to Sweet, 10 November 1942, Box 53, Folder 7, USC Records.

88. See Chapter 6 for further discussion.

89. The UCR Medical Committee included sub-committees for civilian medical services and medical education.

90. Sweet to Edwards, 6 July 1942, Box 53, Folder 10, USC Records.

91. Sweet to Edwards, 31 March 1943, Box 53, Folder 7, USC Records.

92. Forkner to Sweet, 25 May 1943, Box 53, Folder 6, USC Records.

93. Mrs. Edward C. Carter to Van Slyke, 24 February 1944, Box 32, Folder 2, USC Records.

94. Ibid.

95. Soong Ching Ling to Miss Price, 20 September 1943, Box 32, Folder 3, USC Records. Emphasis in original.

96. Ibid.

97. The Ambassador in China (Gauss) to the Secretary of State, 23 February 1944, *Foreign Relations of the United States, 1944, Vol. VI, China* (Washington: GPO, 1947), 352.

98. 9 January 1945, Box 1395, Folder 985.408, RG 200, Records of the American National Red Cross Society.

99. Edwards to Sweet, 7 April 1943, Box 53, Folder 6, USC Records.

100. Williams's projects involved "what he calls first-aid and combat surgery and is confined to training for six weeks to two months." Edwards to Sweet, 7 April 1943, Box 53, Folder 6, USC Records.

Six The Politics of Relief

1. Three examples are Epiphanio Lopez, Alvarez, and Gonzalez. Box 9, Folder 7; Box 8, Folder 13, Martin Papers.

2. Box 9, Folder 26, Martin Papers.

3. Brisker to Martin, 30 June 1969, Box 5, Folder 22, Martin Papers.

4. ARC, 19 August 1942, Box 1, Folder 1, Rose Weiner Papers.

5. Pike had been a chief medical officer with the 15th Brigade. Neugass, *War Is Beautiful*, 85.

6. Klein, Questionnaire, Box 9, Folder 38, Martin Papers.

7. Rose Wachsman Sorkin, Interview, 18–187, John Gerassi Oral History Collection, Tamiment Library, New York University, New York.

8. Leo Eloesser, Questionnaire, Box 7, Folder 11, Martin Papers.

9. Ann X. Smith, "Jersey Nurse Joins UN Organization after Hectic Battle Experience," *Sunday Star-Ledger*, 10 November 1946, Box 1, Folder 5, Patai Papers.

10. Freeman, Questionnaire, Box 8, Folder 7, Martin Papers.

11. Robert W. Clark, "Home from War in Spain, Friedman May Go to China," 13 July 1938, Box 8, Folder 10; "Horrors of Spanish War are Related," Box 10, Folder 17; News Release, Box 5, Folder 3, Martin Papers.

12. Martin to Spiegel, 23 January 1970, Box 8, Folder 18, Martin Papers.

13. Brisker to Martin, 30 June 1969, Box 5, Folder 22, Martin Papers.

14. Byrne to Martin, undated, Box 4, Folder 30, Martin Papers.

15. Grunsky, Questionnaire, Box 8, Folder 33, Martin Papers.

16. Reissig Testimony, 2 May 1939, Box 2, Folder 7, Barsky Papers.

17. Carroll, *Odyssey of the Abraham Lincoln Brigade*, 230. Ironically, the 1818 Neutrality Act also dealt with a matter of Spanish-American relations, albeit inspired by an American who had acted against Spanish sovereignty. Sean T. Perrone, "John Stoughton and the *Divina Pastora* Prize Case, 1816–1818," *Journal of the Early Republic*, 28(2): 2008, 215–241.

18. Carroll, *Odyssey of the Abraham Lincoln Brigade*, 286.

19. Richard O. Boyer, "They're Jailing Anti-Fascists Now," 19 July 1947, Box 5, Folder 14, Martin Papers.

20. Barsky v. Board of Regents 347 U.S. 442, S Ct (1954).

21. Lester to Martin, 25 February 1972, Box 7, Folder 22, Martin Papers.

22. Ena Ferwerda to Martin, 24 January 1970, Box 7, Folder 22, Martin Papers.

23. Interview, Rose Wachsman Sorkin, 18–187, Gerassi Collection.

24. Article, *Holland Herald*, 20–22, Box 6, Folder 14, Martin Papers.

25. Guerra, *La Medicina en el Exilio Republicano*, 524.

26. Song, *Encyclopedia of Chinese-American Relations*, 25–26; Wanda Cornelius and Thayne Short, *Ding Hao: America's Air War in China* (Gretna: Pelican Publishing Company, 2004). For Japan, however, Flying Tiger tactics bordered on banditry and guerrilla warfare, with the threat that any airmen would be treated as such if captured—or, in other words, executed. Webster, *The Burma Road*, 65.

27. "Medicine on a Mission," ABMAC Records.

28. Letter to Mrs. Shipley, 21 January 1937, Box 627, RG 59, General Records of the Department of State.

29. Research conducted by John Earl Haynes and Harvey Klehr could find no official record of a volunteer prosecuted specifically under "premature antifascism", nor any solid historical reference in the numerous studies citing "premature antifascism" or "P.A." as the reason behind later investigations of U.S. veterans of the Spanish Civil War. Harvey Klehr, *The Communist Experience in America: A Political and Social History* (New Brunswick, NJ: Transaction Publishers, 2010), 177–181.

30. This listing associated the CAC as a subsidiary of the American League for Peace and Democracy, also listed as a subversive organization. Committee on Un-American Activities, Guide to Subversive Organizations and Publications, H.R., 2 January 1957.

31. Co Tui, "Plan," 11 April 1939, Box 22, ABMAC Records.

32. Sweet to Edwards, 28 December 1945, Box 51, Folder 6; Edwards to McConaughy, 26 November 1945, Box 51, Folder 7, USC Records.

33. Kohlberg founded the American China Policy Association in 1944 as a means of combating the perceived biases of the Institute of Pacific Relations.

34. Garside to Edwards, 6 June 1947, Box 50, Folder 4, USC Records.

35. Kohlberg to Charles Edison, 20 October 1946, Box 75, Folder 9, USC Records.

36. Ibid.

37. Sweet to Edwards, 26 February 1947, Box 50, Folder 6, USC Records.

38. Edwards to Sweet, 9 September 1947, Box 50, Folder 6, USC Records.

39. Ibid.

40. National Budget Committee to USC, 22 July 1947, Box 18, Folder 8, USC Records.

41. All of this fell under the $1.72 million for UCR's Medical and Public Health Budget. National Budget Committee to USC, 22 July 1947, Box 18, Folder 8, USC Records.

42. "Brief Description of Projects (1948)," Box 16, Folder 18, USC Records.

43. Mildred Price (married name Mildred Coy) was the executive secretary of the China Aid Council in New York. She was also, reportedly, a secret CPUSA member and KGB contact during the Second World War. White Notebook No.2, 9, 33, Box 3; b.4: White Notebook No.3, 105–6, Box 4, Alexander Vassiliev Papers, Manuscript Division, Library of Congress, Washington DC. There is also, according to Haynes, "a January 1946 FBI background file on Mildred Price which notes that the Military Intelligence Division of the War Department had identified Price as an associate of Juliet Poyntz who was an agent of the KGB in the early 1930s and of the GRU in the mid-1930s." (Silvermaster file, 65–56402, serial 356.) "The FBI reports that Duncan Lee, a member of the executive board of the China Aid Council in the early 1940s, was also a secret Communist and, later, a very active Soviet spy when he served as an officer in the Office of Strategic Services." (Sources courtesy of John Earl Haynes, "RE: The China Aid Council" [e-mail to Aelwen Wetherby], 11 August 2011.

44. Sweet to Edwards, 12 July 1946, Box 51, Folder 1, USC Records.

45. R.K.S. Lim to Roger S. Greene, 11 November 1941, Box 22, ABMAC Records.

46. Sweet to Edwards, 16 May 1946, Box 51, Folder 6, USC Records.

47. J. Heng Liu to Kohlberg, 30 March 1943, Box 38, ABMAC Records. Liu was a public health officer with the Nationalist government, who had earned his M.D. at Harvard University and later worked at the PUMC. In October 1946, he became

the ABMAC's medical director in China. Watt, *A Friend in Deed: ABMAC and the Republic of China, 1937–1987.*

48. Joseph Charles Keeley, *The China Lobby Man: The Story of Alfred Kohlberg* (New Rochelle, NY: Arlington House, 1969), 54.

49. "Medicine on a Mission," ABMAC Records.

50. Tae Jin Park, "In Support of 'New China': Origins of the China Lobby, 1937–1941" (unpublished Ph.D. diss., West Virginia University, 2003).

51. Kohlberg to McConnaughy, 28 December 1943, Box 73, Folder 18, USC Records.

52. Apparently Lim did not share Kohlberg's assessment of the situation, and after Kohlberg met with Lim in 1943, Kohlberg wrote, "I had to tell him that he had proven a great disappointment to me . . . All I had been able to get out of him was that the changes were a fait accompli and he had no hard feelings toward anyone." Kohlberg to McConnaughy, 28 December 1943, Box 73, Folder 18, USC Records; ABMAC Reports to Executive Committee, 25 September 1943, Box 3, Folder 12, Opie Papers.

53. This committee consisted of Paul Hoffman, Mr. Henry R. Luce, and Mr. James G. Blaine.

54. Kohlberg to McConnaughy, 21 April 1944, Box 73, Folder 18, USC Records.

55. Kohlberg to Garside, 19 May 1944, Box 73, Folder 18, USC Records.

56. Kohlberg to Van Slyke, 22 December 1943, Box 44, Folder 547, Cannon Papers; Kohlberg to McConnaughy, 28 December 1943, Box 73, Folder 18, USC Records.

57. Inspired, in part, by conversations with ABMAC board member and dentist Maurice Williams, Kohlberg committed himself to an extensive review of IPR coverage of Far Eastern affairs in *Amerasia* alongside a review of two Communist publications—*The New Masses* and *The Communist.* The correlation Kohlberg found between the two led him to conclude that William's suspicions were correct. Keeley, *The China Lobby Man*, 77.

58. Harvey Klehr and Ronald Radosh, *The Amerasia Spy Case: Prelude to McCarthyism* (Chapel Hill: University of North Carolina Press, 1996).

59. Kohlberg's political passions, however, outweighed his religious identity, leading him into close collaboration with Christian Evangelicals and conservative Catholics in the early Cold War period. In setting up a committee to oppose any transfer of American autonomy in foreign policy to a supra-state or international institution, the committee instead recommended that U.S. foreign policy should be based "solidly on Moral Law, Patriotism, Enlightened Nationalism, and the Teachings of Christ." Robert E. Herzstein, "Alfred Kohlberg, Global Entrepeneur and Hyper-Nationalist," presented at the Historical Society, Chapel Hill, NC, 2006, 4–5; Keeley, *The China Lobby Man*, 242–244, 248.

60. Jessica Reinisch, "Internationalism in Relief: The Birth (and Death) of the UNRRA," *Past and Present*, Supplement 6/210 (2011): 258–289.

61. According to Douglas Falconer, deputy director of UNRRA in China: "We, the undersigned, as field service workers for UNRRA, have had the opportunity again and again to see how USC is administering in China the funds entrusted to it by the American public. We have been deeply impressed with the caliber of the personnel, both Chinese and American, in the projects which USC has undertaken to aid and by the harmonious cooperation between them in projects where they are working together." National Budget Committee to USC, 22 July 1947, Box 18, Folder 8, USC Records.

62. Alice Carter to Sweet, 25 February 1947, Box 50, Folder 6, USC Records.

63. "A Special Presentation From American Overseas Aid—UN Appeal for Children," Box 18, Folder 7, USC Records.

64. Victor A. Rule (AOA) to Garside, 10 December 1947, Box 17, Folder 8, USC Records.

65. "The 1949 Program of USC," Box 16, Folder 17, USC Records.

66. "Statement of Policy in Making Appeals for China," Box 21, Folder 6, USC Records.

67. Advertisement, "No Time to Strike Out!" Box 17, Folder 8, USC Records.

68. Ibid.

69. Harry Truman to Lee Marshall, 6 November 1947, Box 18, Folder 7, USC Records.

70. Ibid.

71. "A Proposed Statement of USC's Policy for 1949," Box 21, Folder 6, USC Records.

72. Ibid.

73. Quoted in Donald W. White, *The American Century: The Rise and Decline of the United States as a World Power* (New Haven, CT: Yale University Press, 1996), 211.

74. "Why Is China Important to Us . . . and to the World," Box 21, Folder 6, USC Records.

75. "Meeting—June 1946," Box 21, Folder 6, USC Records. This meeting appears to be the origin for later policy documents that have been cited elsewhere in this section. In these documents, the discussion of the place of democracy in China is conducted in strikingly similar language, while the argument over the place of Western medicine in China is not discussed as directly.

Conclusions

1. Carroll, *Odyssey of the Abraham Lincoln Brigade*, 362.

2. Ibid.

3. Patai, "Eulogy for Fredericka Martin," Box 3, Folder 3, Patai Papers.

4. Patai, "In Memoriam: Rose Wachsman Sorkin (1909–1993)," Box 4, Folder 7, Patai Papers.

5. William P. Coughlin, "Lini De Vries, Teacher, Committed Activist, 76," *Boston Globe,* 1 April 1982, Box 6, Folder 20, Martin Papers.

6. Advertisement, *New York Times*, 2 December 1984, Box 5, Folder 40, Steve Nelson Papers, Tamiment Library, New York University, New York.

7. "Lincoln Brigade Donates Ambulances to Nicaragua," *The Advocate*, 18 April 1985, Box 5, Folder 40, Nelson Papers.

8. Don Duncan, "Spanish War Vets Giving Nicaragua a Hand," *Seattle Times*, 6 March 1985, Box 5, Folder 40, Nelson Papers.

9. Ambulances for Nicaragua, Box 5, Folder 40, Nelson Papers.

10. "Information About Shares, Northwest to Nicaragua Fund Drive," Box 5, Folder 40, Nelson Papers

11. Martin F. Shapiro, "Medical Aid Provided by American, Canadian, and British Nationals to the Spanish Republic During the Civil War, 1936–1939," *International Journal of Health Services* 13 (1983): 443.

12. There remains some unresolved controversy in this group's origins, with historian Stanley Bachrack unable to access CIA records to confirm or negate suspected CIA involvement and support in de Rochefort's earliest petitions. Stanley D. Bachrack, *The Committee of One Million: "China Lobby" Politics, 1953 -1971* (New York: Columbia University Press, 1976), 53.

13. Ibid., 54.

14. Watt, *A Friend in Deed: ABMAC and the Republic of China, 1937–1987*, 10.

15. Ibid., 11.

16. Ibid., 11.

17. Ibid., 114.

18. Garside to R. William Barton, 27 March 1951, Box 70, Folder 11, USC Records.

19. 8 May 1950, Box 73, Folder 18, USC Records.

20. UCR to Advisory Committee on Voluntary Foreign Aid, 15 May 1953, Box 16, Folder 17, USC Records.

21. 3 August 1951, Box 76, Folder 2, USC Records.

22. Anne Vallaeys, *Médecins Sans Frontières: La Biographie* (Paris: Fayard, 2004), 40, 42.

23. Kouchner se refere souvent a l'Espagne republicaine et a l'auteur de l'espoir: "nostalgiques de la guerre d'espagne, nous aurions voulu salver de nos fusils les aviateurs blesses qu'acompagnait Malraux dans la descente de Terruel." Vallaeys, *Médecins Sans Frontières*, 81.

24. Peter Redfield, "A Less Modest Witness: Collective Advocacy and Motivated Truth in a Medical Humanitarian Movement," *American Ethnologist* 33 (2006): 6.

25. Peter Redfield, "Doctors, Borders, and Life in Crisis," *Cultural Anthropology* 20 (2005): 328–361 (329).

26. Ibid., 333.

27. Ibid., 335. For more on Byrne's motivations; see Chapter 1.

28. Redfield, "A Less Modest Witness," 10.

29. Ibid., 3. The Hippocratic Oath reads, "About whatever I may see or hear in treatment, or even without treatment, in the life of human beings—things that

should not ever be blurted out outside—I will remain silent, holding such things to be unutterable."

30. Redfield, "A Less Modest Witness," 3.

31. Taithe, "The Red Cross Flag," 25.

32. Redfield, "A Less Modest Witness," 7.

33. Cannon, "On Medical Aid in Modern War," Box 14, Folder 17, Martin Papers. In addition to his political sympathies, Cannon was also a personal friend of Spanish prime minister Juan Negrín.

34. Which was often even more selectively than the sense of the legal entity of nation-state as sympathies developed for one group within a divided country.

35. Karen Minden, *Bamboo Stone: The Evolution of a Chinese Medical Elite* (Toronto: University of Toronto Press, 1994), 5.

36. Gary Gerstle, *American Crucible: Race and Nation in the Twentieth Century* (Princeton: Princeton University Press, 2002).

37. Edwards to Garside, 15 September 1947, Box 50, Folder 2, USC Records.

38. Edwards to Sweet, 7 August 1947, Box 50, Folder 3, USC Records.

39. "Origins of the AOA," 11, Box 18, Folder 7, USC Records.

40. Dean Acheson to Paul McNutt, 13 April 1949, Box 70, Folder 1, USC Records.

41. Brian Smith, *More Than Altruism: The Politics of Private Aid* (Princeton: Princeton University Press, 1992), 38.

42. Ibid., 37.

43. Office of the Historian, Bureau of Public Affairs, U.S. Department of State, "Lend-Lease and Military Aid to the Allies in the Early Years of World War II," Milestones: 1937–1945, published online at http://history.state.gov/milestones/1937-1945/lend-lease accessed 20 June 2013.

44. Stephen Daggett, "Costs of Major U.S. Wars," Congressional Research Service, 7-5700, RS22926, 29 June 2010, published online at http://www.fas.org/sgp/crs/natsec/RS22926.pdf accessed 20 February 2013.

45. "AOA Questionnaire," 29 October 1947, Box 17, Folder 8, USC Records.

46. "Past Achievements and Present Program," Box 4, Folder 7, USC Records.

47. ABMAC History, Box 1, ABMAC Records.

48. Wilym Jenkins to Edwards, 8 September 1944, Box 53, Folder 1, USC Records.

49. Watt, *A Friend in Deed: ABMAC and the Republic of China, 1937–1987*, 8.

50. Smith, *More Than Altruism*, 41.

51. Box 1395, Folder 985.08, RG 200, Records of the American National Red Cross.

52. Ibid.

53. Ibid.

54. Richard Traina, *American Diplomacy and the Spanish Civil War* (Bloomington: Indiana University Press, 1968).

55. Smith, *American Relief Aid and the Spanish Civil War.*

56. "Statement of Policy in Making Appeals for Support, and Interpreting the Situation in China," Box 21, Folder 6, USC Records.

57. Quoted in David Rieff, "The Wrong Moral Revolution: On Michael Barnett," *The Nation*, 5 October 2011.

58. Ibid.

59. Ultimately, the efforts of the 1930s and 1940s of this study fit much more clearly into Barnett's age of "neo-humanitarianism," whose values share more with nationalism and the Cold War, with an emphasis on development and sovereignty. While a more full reconsideration of his chronological breakdown goes beyond the scope of this study, this author would suggested that using World War II as the tipping point between this new age and the previous (named "imperial humanitarianism" by Barnett) may be misleading, with so much being shared between organizations of the interwar period and those that followed after World War II.

60. Jack C. Fisher and Debra Armstrong, ed., *A Different Kind of Diplomacy: A Source Book for International Health Volunteers* (San Diego, CA: Plastic Surgery Research Foundation, 1987).

61. Ibid.

62. Sparrow, *Warfare State*, 9.

63. Ibid., 11.

Appendix A

1. Guerra, *La Medicina en el Exilio Republicano*, 511–519.

2. Patai cites approximately 25 percent as belonging to the Communist Party. Patai, "Heroines of the Good Fight."

3. Benjamin Segal to Marianne King, 13 October 1937, Box 5, Folder 12, Martin Papers.

4. Helene Weissman, Questionnaire, Box 13, Folder 33, Martin Papers.

5. Alba Novac, Questionnaire, Box 10, Folder 25, Martin Papers.

6. Smith, "New York's Aid," 48.

7. Neugass, *War Is Beautiful.*

8. CSI Pamphlet, Box 5, Folder 21, Martin Papers.

9. Fontaine to Martin, 30 January 1969, Box 7, Folder 24, Martin Papers.

Bibliography

Manuscript and Archival Sources

American Bureau for Medical Aid to China. Records, 1937–1979. Rare Book & Manuscript Library, Columbia University, New York.

American Red Cross. Central File, 1935–1946 (Group 3). National Archive and Records Administration II, College Park, MD.

Barsky, Edward. Papers. Abraham Lincoln Brigade Archives, Tamiment Library, New York University, New York.

Barsky, Edward. Photographs Collection. Abraham Lincoln Brigade Archives, Tamiment Library, New York University, New York.

Cannon, Walter B. Papers. Francis A. Countway Library of Medicine, Harvard University, Boston, MA.

Delano, Frederic A. Papers. Franklin D. Roosevelt Library, Hyde Park, NY.

Foster, John B. Papers. Minnesota Historical Society, St. Paul, MN.

Geiser, Carl. Papers. Abraham Lincoln Brigade Archives, Tamiment Library, New York University, New York.

Gerassi, John. Oral History Collection. Abraham Lincoln Brigade Archives, Tamiment Library, New York University, New York.

Greene, Roger S. Papers. Houghton Library, Harvard University, Boston, MA.

Haskell, Oliver H. Papers. "Oriental Study Expedition Oral History Project." Oral History Collection, Claremont Graduate University, Claremont, CA. Available online at http://web.cgu.edu/oralhistory/pomona_college_oriental_study_expedition.htm.

Hopkins, Harry L. Papers. Franklin D. Roosevelt Library, Hyde Park, NY.

HU 34575—34809. Imperial War Museum Library, London, England.

Jensky, Toby and Philip Schachter. Papers. Abraham Lincoln Brigade Archives, Tamiment Library, New York University, New York.

Landis, Arthur H. Oral History Collection. Abraham Lincoln Brigade Archives, Tamiment Library, New York University, New York.

Lossowski, Vincent. Papers. Abraham Lincoln Brigade Archives, Tamiment Library, New York University, New York.

Martin, Fredericka. Papers. Abraham Lincoln Brigade Archives, Tamiment Library, New York University, New York.

———. Photographs Collection. Abraham Lincoln Brigade Archives, Tamiment Library, New York University, New York.

Nelson, Steve. Papers. Abraham Lincoln Brigade Archives, Tamiment Library, New York University, New York.

Newman, Julia. Papers. Abraham Lincoln Brigade Archives, Tamiment Library, New York University, New York.

Patai, Frances. Papers. Abraham Lincoln Brigade Archives, Tamiment Library, New York University, New York.

———. Photographs Collection. Abraham Lincoln Brigade Archives, Tamiment Library, New York University, New York.

Opie, Eugene. Papers. American Philosophical Society, Philadelphia, PA.

Roosevelt, Franklin D. Papers as President. Franklin D. Roosevelt Library, Hyde Park, NY.

Shafran, Jacob (Jack). Papers. Abraham Lincoln Brigade Archives, Tamiment Library, New York University, New York.

Smith, Randall. Papers. Abraham Lincoln Brigade Archives, Tamiment Library, New York University, New York.

United China Relief. Records, 1928–1947. Manuscripts and Archives Division, New York Public Library, New York.

United Service to China. Records, 1934–1967. Department of Rare Books and Special Collections, Seeley G. Mudd Manuscript Library, Princeton University, Princeton.

Vassiliev, Alexander. Papers. Library of Congress, Manuscript Division, Washington, D.C.

Weiner, Rose. Papers. Abraham Lincoln Brigade Archives, Tamiment Library, New York University, New York.

Wendorf, Paul. Papers. Abraham Lincoln Brigade Archives, Tamiment Library, New York University, New York.

Wilkes, Harry. Papers. Abraham Lincoln Brigade Archives, Tamiment Library, New York University, New York.

Newspapers

The Advocate
Atlanta Constitution
Chicago Daily Tribune
The Chicago Defender
Christian Science Monitor
Hartford Courant
Los Angeles Times
Miami Daily News
The Milwaukee Journal
The New York Times
San Francisco Chronicle
The Seattle Times
The Sun
Washington Post

Printed Primary Sources

"Alumnus Presides over Medical Advancement Program in China." *P&S Journal* 18 (1998).

The Ambassador in China (Gauss) to the Secretary of State, 23 Feb 1944. *Foreign Relations of the United States, 1944, Vol. VI, China.* Washington: GPO, 1947, 352.

Baker, Jay B. "Medical Diplomacy in Full-Spectrum Operations." *Military Review,* Sept–Oct 2007.

Baker, John Earle. *Explaining China.* London: A.M. Philpot Ltd, 1927.

Barsky v. Board of Regents. 347 U.S. 442, S Ct. 1954.

Boardman, Mabel. "Mabel T. Boardman of the American Red Cross on Medical Aid in Modern War." *Journal of the Association of Medical Students,* 1938: 164–165.

Broder, David S. "Diplomacy That Heals." *Washington Post,* 15 January 2009.

Cannon, Walter B. "Walter B. Cannon on Medical Aid in Modern War." *Journal of the Association of Medical Students* (1938).

Cherrington, Ben M. "The Division of Cultural Relations." *Public Opinion Quarterly* 3 (1939) 136–138.

Committee on Un-American Activities, Guide to Subversive Organizations and Publications, H.R., 2 January 1957.

"Congressional Charter of the American National Red Cross." 36 U.S.C. §§300101-300111 recodified 2007. Published online at www.redcross.org/images/pdfs/charter.pdf. Accessed 22 February 2011.

Ewen, Jean. *China Nurse 1932–1939.* Toronto: McClelland and Stewart, 1981.

Freudmann, Dr. W. *Erhebet Euch! Ein Arzt Erlebt China.* Verlag, Linz-Urfahr: Neue Zeit, 1947.

Garside, B.A. *Within the Four Seas.* New York: Frederic C. Beil, 1985.

Hemenway, Ruth V. *Ruth V. Hemenway, M.D.: A Memoir of Revolutionary China, 1924–1941.* Amherst: University of Massachusetts Press, 1977.

Jensen, Fritz. *China Siegt.* Wien: Stern, 1949.

Malbin, Barney. "Typhoid Fever Occurring in Immunized Persons." *The Journal of the American Medical Association* 115 (1940): 33–36.

Mr. Lauchlin Currie to President Roosevelt, 15 March 1941. *Foreign Relations of the United States, 1944, Vol. VI, China.* Washington: GPO, 1947, 94.

Neugass, James. *War Is Beautiful: An American Ambulance Driver in the Spanish Civil War.* Edited by Peter N. Carroll and Peter Glazer. New York: New Press, 2008.

O'Reilly, Salaria Kee. "While Passing Through." *Health & Medicine* 4/1 (Spring 1987): 11–13.

Orwell, George. *Homage to Catalonia.* Orlando: Harcourt, 1952.

Roosevelt, Franklin Delano. "Executive Order 9205 Establishing the President's War Relief Control Board." July 25, 1942. Published online by *The American Presidency Project.* Edited by Gerhard Peters and John T. Woolley. http://www.presidency.ucsb.edu/ws/?pid=16287.

President Roosevelt to the Secretary of State and to the Chairman of the American National Red Cross, 11 Jan 1938. Foreign Relations of the United States, 1938, Vol. IV: The Far East. Washington: GPO, 1954, 571.

———. "Radio Address on the National War Fund." 5 October 1943. Published online by *The American Presidency Project.* Edited by Gerhard Peters and John T. Woolley. http://www.presidency.ucsb.edu/ws/index.php?pid=16322.

Rubin, Hank. *Spain's Cause Was Mine: A Memoir of an American Medic in the Spanish Civil War.* Carbondale, IL: Southern Illinois University Press, 1997.

Seagrave, Gordon Stiffler. *Burma Surgeon.* London: V. Gollancz Ltd., 1944.

Simpson, John E. *Letters from China: Quaker Relief Work in Bandit Country, 1944–1946* Cambridge, UK: Ross-Evans, 2001.

Stanley, Margaret. "China: Then and Now." *American Journal of Nursing* 72 (1972): 2213–2218.

———. "Two Experiences of an American Public Health Nurse in China a Quarter of a Century Apart." *American Journal of Public Health* 63 (1973): 111–116.

Thompson, Donald F. "The Role of Medical Diplomacy in Stabilizing Afghanistant," *Defense Horizons,* No. 63, May 2008.

Thompson, Tommy G. "The Cure for Tyranny." *Boston Globe,* 24 October 2005.

Printed Secondary Works

Allan, Ted, and Gordon, Sydney. *The Scalpel, the Sword: The Story of Dr. Norman Bethune.* New York: Monthly Review Press, 1973.

Bachrack, Stanley D. *The Committee of One Million: "China Lobby" Politics, 1953–1971.* New York: Columbia University Press, 1976.

Bailey, Sydney D. "Review of Quaker Relief: An Account of the Relief Work of the Society of Friends." *International Affairs* 29 (1953): 270.

Balogh, Brian. *A Government Out of Sight: The Mystery of National Authority in Nineteenth Century America.* Cambridge: Cambridge University Press, 2009.

Barnett, Michael. *Empire of Humanity: A History of Humanitarianism.* Ithaca: Cornell University Press, 2011.

———, and Weiss, Thomas George. *Humanitarianism Contested: Where Angels Fear to Tread.* Milton Park, England: Routledge, 2011.

———, and Weiss, Thomas George, eds. *Humanitarianism in Question: Politics, Power, Ethics.* Ithaca: Cornell University Press, 2008.

Barona Vilar, Josep Lluís. "Negrín medico fisiólogo." *Juan Negrín Médico y Jefe de Gobierno, 1892–1956.* Madrid: Minesterio de Cultura, SECC, 2006.

———. "Nutrition and Health: The International Context during the Inter-War Crisis." *Social History of Medicine* 21/1 (2008): 87–105.

———. "The Rockefeller Foundation, Social Policies and Public Health in Spain, 1920–1939," in *American Foundations and the European Welfare States.* Odense: University Press of Southern Denmark, 2013.

———. *Salud, Enfermedad y Muerte: La Sociedad Valenciana Entre 1833 y 1939.* Valencia: Institucio Alfons El Magnanim, 2002.

———, and Perdiguero-Gil, Enrique. "Health and the War. Changing Schemes and Health Conditions During the Spanish Civil War." *Dynamis* 28 (2008): 103–126.

Baudendistel, Rainer. *Between Bombs and Good Intentions: The Red Cross and the Italo-Ethiopian War, 1935–1936.* New York: Berghahn Books, 2006.

Bender, Thomas. *A Nation among Nations: America's Place in World History.* New York: Hill & Wang, 2006.

Benison, Saul, Barger, Clifford A., and Wolfe, Elin L. "Walter B. Cannon and the Mystery of Shock: A Study of Anglo-American Cooperation in World War I." *Medical History* 35 (1991).

Bolling, Landrum R., and Smith, Craig. *Private Foreign Aid: U.S. Philanthropy for Relief and Development.* Boulder, CO: Westview Press, 1982.

Brandt, Allan M. *No Magic Bullet: A Social History of Venereal Disease in the United States Since 1880.* New York: Oxford University Press, 1985.

Bremner, Robert H. *American Philanthropy.* Chicago: University of Chicago Press, 1988.

Brinkley, Alan. *The Publisher: Henry Luce and His American Century.* New York: Alfred A. Knopf, 2010.

Buchanan, Tom. *Britain and the Spanish Civil War.* Cambridge: Cambridge University Press, 1997.

———. "Britain's Popular Front?: Aid Spain and the British Labour Movement." History Workshop Journal 31/1 (1991): 60-72.

———. *East Wind: China and the British Left, 1925–1976* (Oxford: Oxford University Press, 2012).

———. *The Impact of the Spanish Civil War on Britain: War, Loss and Memory.* Brighton: Sussex Academic Press, 2007.

———. "Review of Angela Jackson, British Women and the Spanish Civil War." H-Albion, *H-Net Reviews,* September 2003. Published online at http://www.h-net.org/reviews/showrev.cgi?path=275351068285472.

———. "'Shanghai-Madrid Axis'? Comparing British Responses to the Conflicts in Spain and China, 1936–1949." *Contemporary European History* 21 (2012): 533–552.

Bullock, Mary Brown. *An American Transplant: The Rockefeller Foundation and Peking Union Medical College.* Berkeley: University of California Press, 1980.

Cabanes, Bruno. *The Great War and the Origins of Humanitarianism, 1918–1924.* Cambridge: Cambridge University Press, 2014.

Carroll, Peter N. *The Odyssey of the Abraham Lincoln Brigade: Americans in the Spanish Civil War.* Palo Alto, CA: Stanford University Press, 1994.

Celada, Antonio R., García, Daniel Pastor, and López Alonso, Rosa María, eds. *Las Brigadas Internacionales: 70 Años de Memoria Histórica.* Salamanca: Amarú Ediciones, 2007.

Cohen, Warren I. *America's Response to China: An Interpretive History of Sino-American Relations*. New York: John Wiley & Sons, Inc., 1971.

———. *Empire without Tears: America's Foreign Relations, 1921–1933*. New York: Alfred A. Knopf, 1987.

Collum, Danny Duncan, ed. *African Americans in the Spanish Civil War: "This Ain't Ethiopia, But It'll Do."* New York: G.K. Hall, 1992.

Coni, Nicolas. *Medicine and Warfare: Spain, 1936–1939*. New York: Routledge, 2008.

Cornelius, Wanda, and Short, Thayne. *Ding Hao: America's Air War in China*. Gretna: Pelican Publishing Company, 2004.

Cowdrey, Albert E. *Fighting for Life: American Military Medicine in World War II*. New York: Free Press, 1994.

Curti, Merle. *American Philanthropy Abroad*. New Brunswick, NJ: Rutgers University Press, 1963.

Dallek, Robert. *Franklin D. Roosevelt and American Foreign Policy, 1932–1945*. Oxford, Oxford University Press, 1995.

Davenport, Horace W. *Robert Kho-Seng Lim, 1897–1969*. Washington D.C.: The National Academies Press, 1980.

Davies, A. Tegla. *Friends Ambulance Unit: The Story of the F.A.U. in the Second World War 1939–1946*. London: George Allen and Unwin Limited, 1947.

Del Cura, María Isabel, and Huertas, Rafael. *Alimentación y Enfermedad En Tiempos De Hambre, España, 1937–1947*. Madrid: Consejo Superior de Investigaciones Científicas, 2007.

Dulles, Foster Rhea. *The American Red Cross: A History*. Westport, CT: Greenwood Press, 1950.

Epstein, Israel. *Woman in World History: Life and Times of Soong Ching Ling (Mme. Sun Yatsen)*. Beijing: Foreign Languages Press, 2004.

Fisher, Jack C., and Armstrong, Debra, eds. *A Different Kind of Diplomacy: A Source Book for International Health Volunteers*. San Diego, CA: Plastic Surgery Research Foundation, 1987.

Foner, Eric, and McGirr, Lisa, eds. *American History Now: Critical Perspectives on the Past*. Philadelphia: Temple University Press, 2011.

Forsythe, David P. *The Humanitarians: The International Committee of the Red Cross*. Cambridge: Cambridge University Press, 2005.

Fyrth, Jim. *The Signal Was Spain: The Spanish Aid Movement in Britain, 1936–1939*. London: Lawrence & Wishart, 1986.

Gerstle, Gary. *American Crucible: Race and Nation in the Twentieth Century*. Princeton: Princeton University Press, 2002.

Guerra, Francisco. *La Medicina en el Exilio Republicano*. Madrid: Universidad de Alcala de Henares, 2003.

Guttman, Allen. *The Wound in the Heart: America and the Spanish Civil War*. New York: Free Press, 1962.

Hammack, David C. "Failure and Resilience: Pushing the Limits in Depression and Wartime." In *Charity, Philanthropy, and Civility in American History*. Edited by Lawrence J. Friedman and Mark D. McGarvie. Cambridge, UK: Cambridge University Press, 2003.

Hannant, Larry. *The Politics of Passion: Norman Bethune's Writing and Art.* Toronto: University of Toronto Press, 1998.

Harrison, Mark. *The Medical War: British Military Medicine in the First World War.* Oxford: Oxford University Press, 2010.

———. "The Medicalization of War—The Militarization of Medicine." *Social History of Medicine* 9 (1996): 267–276.

———. "Medicine and the Management of Modern Warfare." History of Science 34 (1996): 379-410.

Herrick, Claire. "'The Conquest of the Silent Foe': British and American Military Medical Reform Rhetoric and the Russo-Japanese War." In *Medicine and Modern Warfare.* Edited by Roger Cooter, Mark Harrison, and Steve Sturdy. Amsterdam: Rodopi, 1999.

Hervás, C., and Unzueta, M. "Robert Macintosh and the Spanish Civil War: A New Perspective." *International Congress Series* 1242 (2002): 411–420.

Hsu, Madeline Y. "Befriending the Yellow Peril: Student Migration and the Warming of American Attitudes Toward Chinese, 1905–1950." In *Trans-Pacific Interactions: The United States and China, 1880–1950.* Edited by Vanessa Künnemann and Ruth Mayer. New York: Palgrave Macmillan, 2009.

Huber, Max. *The Red Cross: Principles and Problems, 1939–1946.* Geneva: A. Kundig, 1947.

Humphreys, George H., II. "An Early Contact Between the Columbia University College of Physicians and Surgeons and National Taiwan University: Two Accounts." In *Health Care and National Development in Taiwan, 1950–2000.* Edited By John Watt. New York: ABMAC Foundation, 2008.

Hunter, Alan, and Kim-Kwong, Chan. *Protestantism in Contemporary China.* Cambridge: Cambridge University Press, 1993.

Hutchinson, John F. *Champions of Charity: War and the Rise of the Red Cross.* Boulder: Westview Press, 1996.

———. "'Custodians of the Sacred Fire': The International Committee of the Red Cross and the Postwar Reorganisation of the International Red Cross." In *International Health Organisations and Movements, 1918–1939.* Edited by Paul Weindling. Cambridge: Cambridge University Press, 1995.

Iriye, Akira. *China and Japan in the Global Setting.* Cambridge, MA: Harvard University Press, 1992.

———. *Cultural Internationalism and World Order.* Baltimore: Johns Hopkins University Press, 1997.

———. *Global Community: The Role of International Organizations in the Making of the Contemporary World.* Berkeley: University of California Press, 2002.

———. "The Internationalization of History." *American Historical Review* 94 (1989): 1–10.

———. "The Role of International Organizations." In *The Global History Reader.* Edited by Bruce Mazlish and Akira Iriye. New York: Routledge, 2005.

Irwin, Julia. *Making the World Safe: The American Red Cross and a Nation's Humanitarian Awakening.* Oxford: Oxford University Press, 2013.

Israel, Jerry. "Carl Crow, Edgar Snow, and Shifting American Journalistic Perceptions of China." In *America Views China: American Images of China Then and Now.* Bethlehem, PA: Lehigh University Press, 1991.

Jackson, Angela. *At the Margins of Mayhem.* Pontypool: Warren & Pell Publishing, 2008.

———. *Beyond the Battlefield: Testimony, Memory, and Remembrance of a Cave Hospital.* Pontypool: Warren & Pell Publishing, 2005.

———. *British Women and the Spanish Civil War.* London: Routledge, 2002.

———. *For Us it Was Heaven: The Passion, Grief & Fortitude of Patience Darton—from the Spanish Civil War to Mao's China.* Sussex: Sussex Academic Press, 2012.

Jackson, Gabriel. *Juan Negrín: Spanish Republican War Leader.* Sussex: Sussex Academic Press, 2010.

———. *The Spanish Republic and the Civil War, 1931–1939.* Princeton: Princeton University Press, 1965.

Jespersen, T. Christopher. *American Images of China, 1931–1949.* Stanford, CA: Stanford University Press, 1996.

Jones, Marian Moser. *The American Red Cross from Clara Barton to the New Deal.* Baltimore: Johns Hopkins University Press, 2013.

Keeley, Joseph Charles. *The China Lobby Man: The Story of Alfred Kohlberg.* New Rochelle, NY: Arlington House, 1969.

King, Betty L. "Memories of Dr. Frank Co Tui: Physician, Scientist (1897–1984)." In *Health Care and National Development in Taiwan.* New York: ABMAC Foundation, 2008.

Klehr, Harvey. *The Communist Experience in America: A Political and Social History.* New Brunswick, NJ: Transaction Publishers, 2010.

———, and Radosh, Ronald. *The Amerasia Spy Case: Prelude to McCarthyism.* Chapel Hill: University of North Carolina Press, 1996.

Künnemann, Vanessa. "'Following with Bleeding Footsteps?' American Missions in China and the (Gendered) Critique of Pearl S. Buck." In *Trans-Pacific Interactions: The United States and China, 1880–1950.* Edited by Vanessa Künnemann and Ruth Mayer. New York: Palgrave Macmillan, 2009.

Lee, Edwards. *Missionary for Freedom: The Life and Times of Walter Judd.* New York: Paragon House, 1990.

Leong, Karen J. *The China Mystique: Pearl S. Buck, Anna May Wong, Mayling Soong, and the Transformation of American Orientalism.* Berkeley: University of California Press, 2005.

Li, Cheng. "Coming Home to Teach: Status and Mobility of Returnees in China's Higher Education." In *Bridging Minds across the Pacific: U.S.-China Educational Exchanges, 1978–2003.* Edited by Cheng Li. Lanham, MD: Lexington Books, 2005.

Link, Eugene Perry. *The Social Ideas of American Physicians (1776–1976): Studies in the Humanitarian Tradition of Medicine.* London: Associated University Presses, 1992.

Love, Spencie. *One Blood: The Death and Resurrection of Charles R. Drew.* Chapel Hill: University of North Carolina Press, 1997.

Madero, Manuel Olarte. *Las Brigadas Internacionales: El "Hospital Inglés De Huete."* Cuenca: Imprenta Rápida Conquense, 2010.

Manela, Erez. *The Wilsonian Moment: Self-Determination and the International Origins of Anticolonial Nationalism.* Oxford: Oxford University Press, 2007.

Massons, José M. *Historia de la Sanidad Militar Española, Tomo II.* Barcelona: Ediciones Pomares-Corredor, 1994.

McKean, David. *Peddling Influence: Thomas "Tommy the Cork" Corcoran and the Birth of Modern Lobbying.* Hanover, NH: Steerforth, 2005.

Merrill, Dennis, and Paterson, Thomas G., eds. *Major Problems in American Foreign Relations: Documents and Essays.* 7th ed. 2 vols. Boston: Wadsworth Cengage Learning, 2010.

Minden, Karen. *Bamboo Stone: The Evolution of a Chinese Medical Elite.* Toronto: University of Toronto Press, 1994.

Miscevic, Dusanka, and Kwong, Peter. *Chinese Americans: The Immigrant Experience.* Southport, CT: Hugh Lauter Levin Associates, Inc., 2000.

Mitter, Rana. *A Bitter Revolution: China's Struggle with the Modern World.* Oxford: Oxford University Press, 2004.

Molesworth, Carl. *Sharks over China: The 23rd Fighter Group in World War II.* Washington D.C.: Brassey's, 1994.

Navarro Carballo, José Ramón. *La Sanidad en las Brigadas Internacionales.* Madrid: Servicio de Publicaciones del Estado Mayor del Ejercito, 1989.

Neils, Patricia. *China Images in the Life and Times of Henry Luce.* Savage, MD: Rowman & Littlefield Publishers, Inc., 1990.

Nelson, Cary, and Hendricks, Jefferson, eds. *Madrid 1937: Letters of the Abraham Lincoln Brigade from the Spanish Civil War.* New York: Routledge, 1996.

Palfreeman, Linda. *¡Salud! British Volunters in the Republican Medical Service During the Spanish Civil War, 1936–1939.* Eastbourne: Sussex Academic Press, 2012.

Patai, Frances. "Heroines of the Good Fight: Testimonies of U.S. Volunteer Nurses in the Spanish Civil War, 1936–1939." *Nursing History Review* 3 (1995): 79–104.

Patenaude, Bertrand M. *The Big Show in Bololand: The American Relief Expedition to Soviet Russia in the Famine of 1921.* Palo Alto, CA: Stanford University Press, 2002.

Perrone, Sean T. "John Stoughton and the *Divina Pastora* Prize Case, 1816–1818." *Journal of the Early Republic* 28/2 (2008): 215–241.

Pfaelzer, Jean. *Driven Out: The Forgotten War against Chinese Americans.* Berkeley: University of California Press, 2008.

Plummer, Brenda Gayle. "The Changing Face of Diplomatic History: A Literature Review." *The History Teacher* 38 (2005): 385–400.

Redfield, Peter. "A Less Modest Witness: Collective Advocacy and Motivated Truth in a Medical Humanitarian Movement." *American Ethnologist* 33/1 (2006): 3–26.

———. "Doctors, Borders, and Life in Crisis." *Cultural Anthropology* 20/3 (2005): 328–361.

Reeves, Caroline. "From Red Crosses to Golden Arches: China, the Red Cross, and the Hague Peace Conference, 1899–1900." In *Interactions: Transregional Perspectives on World History*. Edited by Jerry H. Bentley, Renate Bridenthal, and Anand A. Yang. Honolulu: University of Hawaii Press, 2005.

Reinisch, Jessica. "Internationalism in Relief: The Birth (and Death) of the UNRRA," *Past and Present*, Supplement 6/210 (2011): 258–289.

———. *The Perils of Peace: The Public Health Crisis in Occupied Germany*. Oxford: Oxford University Press, 2013.

———, and Elizabeth White. *The Disentanglement of Populations: Migration, Expulsion and Displacement in Postwar Europe, 1944–49*. Basingstoke: Palgrave Macmillan, 2011.

———, Mazower, Mark, and Feldman, David, eds. *Post-War Reconstruction in Europe: International Perspectives, 1945–1949*. Oxford: Oxford University Press, 2011.

Requena, Manuel and Mª Sepúlveda, Rosa, eds. *La Sanidad en las Brigadas Internacionales*. Cuenca: Ediciones de la Universidad de Castilla-La Mancha, 2006.

Rey García, Marta. *Stars for Spain: La Guerra Civil Española en los Estados Unidos*. Madrid: Edició́s de Castro, 1995.

Rieff, David. "The Wrong Moral Revolution: On Michael Barnett." *The Nation*, 5 October 2011.

Rosenberg, Emily S. "Missions to the World: Philanthropy Abroad." In *Charity, Philanthropy, and Civility in American History*. Edited by Lawrence J. Friedman and Mark D. McGarvie. Cambridge: Cambridge University Press, 2003.

———. *Spreading the American Dream: American Economic and Cultural Expansion, 1890–1945*. New York: Hill & Wang, 1982.

Ross, Red. "Black Americans and Italo-Ethiopian Relief 1935–1936." In *Race and U.S. Foreign Policy from the Colonial Period to the Present*. Edited by Michael Krenn. London: Routledge, 1998.

Schaller, Michael. *The U.S. Crusade in China, 1938–1945*. New York: Columbia University Press, 1979.

———. *The United States and China: Into the Twenty-First Century*. New York: Oxford University Press, 2002.

Selverstone, Marc J. "A Literature So Immense: The Historiography of Anticommunism." *OAH Magazine of History* 24 (2010): 7–11.

Seymour, Harold J. *Design for Giving: The Story of the National War Fund, Inc., 1943–1947*. New York: Harper & Brothers, 1947.

Shapiro, Martin F. "Medical Aid Provided by American, Canadian and British Nationals to the Spanish Republic During the Civil War, 1936–1939." *International Journal of Health Services* 13/3 (1983): 443–458.

Shapiro, Sidney. *Ma Haide: The Saga of American Doctor George Hatem in China*. Beijing: Foreign Languages Press, 2004.

Shealy, Gwendolyn C. *A Critical History of the American Red Cross, 1882–1945: The End of Noble Humanitarianism*. Lewiston, NY: Edwin Mellen Press, 2003.

Shephard, Ben. *The Long Road Home: The Aftermath of the Second World War*. London: Vintage Books, 2012.

Shewmaker, Kenneth E. *Americans and Chinese Communists, 1927–1945: A Persuading Encounter*. Ithaca: Cornell University Press, 1971.

Shumaker, Harris B. *Leo Eloesser, M.D.: Eulogy for a Free Spirit*. New York: Philosophical Library, 1982.

Sichon, G.E. "Mémoires et témoignages, Les médicins des deux guerres: Espagne 1936–1939, Chine 1939–1945." *Matériaux pour l'histoire de notre temps* 19 (1990): 57–64.

Smith, Brian. *More Than Altruism: The Politics of Private Aid*. Princeton: Princeton University Press, 1992.

Smith, Eric R. *American Relief Aid and the Spanish Civil War*. Columbia: University of Missouri Press, 2013.

———. "New York's Aid to the Spanish Republic." In *Facing Fascism: New York and the Spanish Civil War*. Edited by Peter N. Carroll and James D. Fernández. New York: New York University Press, 2007.

Song, Yuwu, ed. *Encyclopedia of Chinese-American Relations*. Jefferson, NC: McFarland & Co., 2006.

Sparrow, James T. *Warfare State: World War II Americans and the Age of Big Government*. New York: Oxford University Press, 2011.

Spence, Jonathan D. *The Search for Modern China*. New York: W. W. Norton & Company, 1990.

Stewart, Roderick, and Stewart, Sharon. *Phoenix: The Life of Norman Bethune*. Montreal: McGill-Queens University Press, 2012.

Stuhler, Barbara. "Review of Missionary for Freedom: The Life and Times of Walter Judd." *Minnesota History* 52 (1991): 200.

Taithe, Bertrand. "The Red Cross Flag in the Franco-Prussian War: Civilians, Humanitarians and War in the 'Modern Age.'" In *War, Medicine and Modernity*. Edited by Roger Cooter, Mark Harrison, and Steve Sturdy. Stroud: Sutton Publishing, 1998.

Thomas, Hugh. *The Spanish Civil War*. 4th ed. London: Penguin, 2003.

Thomas, Jose Maria. *Roosevelt and Franco During the Second World War: From the Spanish Civil War to Pearl Harbor*. New York: Palgrave Macmillan, 2008.

Thomson, James C., Jr., *While China Faced West: American Reformers in Nationalist China, 1928–1937*. Cambridge, MA: Harvard University Press, 1969.

Tierney, Dominic. *FDR and the Spanish Civil War: Neutrality and Commitment in the Struggle That Divided America*. Durham, NC: Duke University Press, 2007.

Towers, Bridget. "Red Cross Organisational Politics, 1918–1922: Relations of Dominance and the Influence of the United States." In *International Health Organisations and Movements, 1918–1939*. Edited by Paul Weindling. Cambridge: Cambridge University Press, 1995.

Traina, Richard. *American Diplomacy and the Spanish Civil War*. Bloomington: Indiana University Press, 1968.

Tuchman, Barbara W. *Stilwell and the American Experience in China, 1911–1945*. New York: Macmillan Company, 1971.

Tusan, Michelle. *Smyrna's Ashes: Humanitarianism, Genocide, and the Birth of the Middle East*. Berkeley: University of California Press, 2012.

Tyrrell, Ian. *Reforming the World: The Creation of America's Moral Empire*. Princeton: Princeton University Press, 2010.

———. *Transnational Nation: United States history in Global Perspective Since 1789*. Basingstoke, UK: Palgrave Macmillan, 2007.

———. *Woman's World, Woman's Empire: The Woman's Christian Temperance Union in International Perspective, 1880–1930*. Chapel Hill: University of North Carolina Press, 1991.

Vallaeys, Anne. *Médecins Sans Frontières: La Biographie*. Paris: Fayard, 2004.

Wang, Y.S., and Cheng, T.O. "Leo Eloesser: An American Cardiothoracic Surgeon in China." *Annals of Thoracic Surgery* 71 (2001): 1387–1388.

Watenpaugh, Keith David. *Bread from Stones: The Middle East and the Making of Modern Humanitarianism*. Oakland: University of California Press, 2015.

Watt, John R. *A Friend in Deed: ABMAC and the Republic of China, 1937–1987*. New York: ABMAC Foundation, 1992.

———, ed. *Health Care and National Development in Taiwan, 1950–2000*. New York: ABMAC Foundation, 2008.

Webster, Donovan. *The Burma Road: The Epic Story of One of World War II's Most Remarkable Endeavours*. London: Macmillan, 2003.

Weindling, Paul, ed. *International Health Organisations and Movements, 1918–1939*. Cambridge: Cambridge University Press, 1995.

White, Donald W. *The American Century: The Rise and Decline of the United States as a World Power*. New Haven, CT: Yale University Press, 1996.

Wiesmann, William, Draghic, Nicole, and Parrish, John A. "Advances in Modern Combat Casualty Care With a Vision to the Future." *In War and Medicine*. Edited by the Wellcome Trust. London: Black Dog, 2008, 227–241.

Wolfe, Elin L., Barger, Clifford A., and Benison, Saul. *Walter B. Cannon: Science and Society*. Cambridge, MA: Harvard University Press, 2000.

Yu, Maochun. *OSS in China: Prelude to Cold War*. Annapolis: Naval Institute Press, 2011.

Zunz, Olivier. *Philanthropy in America: A History*. Princeton: Princeton University Press, 2011.

Unpublished Dissertations

Brewer, Karen Lynn. "From Philanthropy to Reform: The American Red Cross in China, 1906–1930." PhD diss., Case Western Reserve University, 1983.

Guptil, Marilla Bliss. "The United States and Foreign Relief: UNRRA in China, 1942–1947." PhD diss., University of Virginia, 1995.

Heavens, John. "The International Committee of the North American Young Men's Christian Association and Its Foreign Work in China, 1895–1937." PhD diss., University of Cambridge, 2013.

Irwin, Julia. "Humanitarian Occupations: Foreign Relief and Assistance in the Formation of American International Identities, 1898–1928." PhD diss., Yale University, 2009.

Jones, Marian Moser. "Confronting Calamity: The American Red Cross and the Politics of Disaster Relief, 1881–1939." PhD diss., Columbia University, 2008.

Mendlesohn, F. "Practising Peace: American and British Quaker Relief in the Spanish Civil War." DPhil diss., University of York, 1997.

Park, Tae Jin. "In Support of 'New China': Origins of the China Lobby, 1937–1941." PhD diss., West Virginia University, 2003.

Reeves, Caroline. "The Power of Mercy: The Chinese Red Cross Society, 1900–1937." PhD diss., Harvard University, 1998.

Reynolds, Thomas H. "American Red Cross Disaster Services, 1930–1947." PhD diss., Columbia University, 1954.

Smith, Eric R. "Anti-fascism, the United Front, and Spanish Republican Aid in the United States, 1936–1940." PhD diss., University of Illinois at Chicago, 2007. [Author's copy electronic rtf file, courtesy of Eric R. Smith.]

Thompson, Eleanor. "Social Reconstructionism: An Intellectual History of Radicalism in American Education from the Progressive Era to the New Deal." DPhil diss., University of Oxford, 2011.

Other Sources

The American Red Cross. "100 Significant Dates in Red Cross History." Published online at http://www.redcross.org/museum/history/100dates.asp. Accessed 22 February 2011.

Andres, Josefa. Interview by Dorothy Eubanks and Aelwen Wetherby. Translated by Aelwen Wetherby, 2012.

Biographical on Marian Yang courtesy of the research notes of Dr. Nicole Barnes, shared via e-mail 27 June 2013. (Based on research conducted at Rockefeller Foundation Archives in Tarrytown, New York.)

The Charles R. Drew Papers, Profiles in Medicine, National Library of Medicine. "Plasma for Great Britain." Published online at http://profiles.nlm.nih.gov/BG/. Accessed on 22 May 2013.

Daggett, Stephen. "Costs of Major U.S. Wars." Congressional Research Service, 7–5700, RS22926, 29 June 2010. Published online at http://www.fas.org/sgp/crs/natsec/RS22926.pdf. Accessed 20 February 2013.

Falo, Juana Barreras. Interview by Dorothy Eubanks and Aelwen Wetherby. Translated by Aelwen Wetherby, 2012.

Herzstein, Robert E. "Alfred Kohlberg, Global Entrepeneur and Hyper-Nationalist." Presented at the Historical Society, Chapel Hill, NC: 2006.

Newman, Julia, dir. *Into the Fire: American Women in the Spanish Civil War.* First Run Features, 2002.

Reeves, Caroline. "History of the Chinese Red Cross: Part II." China Beat. http://www.thechinabeat.org/?p=119. Last modified 20 May 2008. Accessed 22 February 2011.

Tsang, Steve. "Chiang Kai-shek's 'Secret Deal' at Xian and the Start of the Sino-Japanese War." *Palgrave Communications* 1. Published online 20 January 2015. http://www.palgrave-journals.com/articles/palcomms20143.

Index

Page references in italics are to illustrations.